First Strike

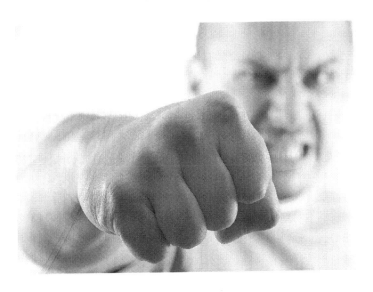

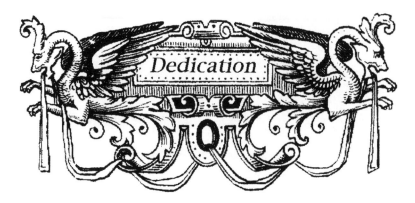

Dedication

For Fonto

First Strike

End a Fight in Ten Seconds or Less!

SAMMY FRANCO

Also by Sammy Franco

Kubotan Power
The Complete Body Opponent Bag Book
Heavy Bag Training: Boxing, Mixed Martial Arts & Self-Defense
Gun Safety: For Home Defense and Concealed Carry
Out of the Cage: A Complete Guide to Beating a Mixed Martial Artist on the Street
Warrior Wisdom: Inspiring Ideas from the World's Greatest Warriors
Judge, Jury and Executioner
Savage Street Fighting: Tactical Savagery as a Last Resort
Feral Fighting: Level 2 WidowMaker
War Craft: Street Fighting Tactics of the War Machine
War Machine: How to Transform Yourself Into a Vicious and Deadly Street Fighter
The Bigger They Are, The Harder They Fall: How to Defeat a Larger & Stronger Adversary in a Street Fight
1001 Street Fighting Secrets: The Principles of Contemporary Fighting Arts
When Seconds Count: Everyone's Guide to Self-Defense
Killer Instinct: Unarmed Combat for Street Survival
Street Lethal: Unarmed Urban Combat

First Strike: End a Fight in Ten Seconds or Less!
Copyright © 2014 by Sammy Franco
ISBN 978-0-9853472-8-4
Printed in the United States of America

Published by Contemporary Fighting Arts, LLC.
P.O. Box 84028
Gaithersburg, Maryland 20883 USA
Phone: (301) 279-2244
Visit us Online at: www.sammyfranco.com

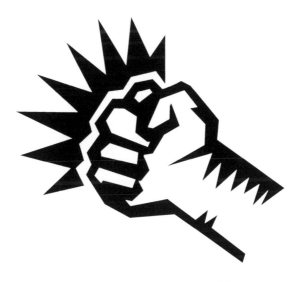

Rear Web-Hand Strike
Rear Horizontal Elbow
Rear Diagonal Elbow
Advanced First-Strike Tools

Hook Kick
Lead Straight
Rear Cross
Lead Hook Punch
Rear Hook Punch
Lead Uppercut
Rear Uppercut
Lead Shovel Hook
Rear Shovel Hook
Rear Vertical Hammer Fist
Rear Vertical Knee
Rear Diagonal Knee
Continual Practice Is Essential
Training Routines

First-Strike Scenarios
Advanced Scenarios
Makeshift-Weapon Scenario

"When danger is imminent, strike first, strike fast, strike with authority, and keep the pressure on."

- Sammy Franco (1982)

ACKNOWLEDGMENTS

Special thanks to the people throughout the world for their support, interest, and loyalty to my system of self-defense - Contemporary Fighting Arts.

ABOUT THIS BOOK

This book is designed to instruct you in the art and science of launching a preemptive strike in a self-defense situation. To the best of my knowledge, no text has been written about this critical, yet often overlooked, aspect of self-defense. This book that you are holding in your hands is truly the first of its kind.

The contents of this text will undoubtedly provide you with the where-withal to effectively execute a first strike and ultimately prevail in a volatile confrontation. Beware, the information and techniques contained herein are dangerous and should only be used to protect yourself or a loved one from the immediate risk of unlawful injury. Remember, the decision to launch a first strike must always be a last resort, after all other means of avoiding violence have been exhausted.

This text is both a skill-building workbook and strategic blueprint for combat. Feel free to write in the margins, underline passages, and dog-ear the pages. I strongly recommend that you read this text from beginning to end, chapter by chapter. Only after you have read the entire book should you treat it like a reference and skip around, reading those sections that interest you.

Finally, at the end of this book I have included two appendices that should be closely studied. In addition, since most of the words in this text are defined within the context of Contemporary Fighting Arts and its related elements, I have provided a glossary.

Sammy Franco,
Founder and President
Contemporary Fighting Arts

CONTEMPORARY FIGHTING ARTS
NO BELTS - NO RITUALS - NO NONSENSE

All the concepts, principles, and terms in this book are based on the teachings of Contemporary Fighting Arts (CFA). I'm not going to spend a lot of time in this book describing CFA to you because it has been covered in my previous books. However, for those who have not read any of my previous books, I would like to provide a brief overview of what CFA is.

Contemporary Fighting Arts is a reality based self-defense system designed specifically to provide the most efficient and effective methods possible to avoid, defuse, confront, and neutralize both armed and unarmed opponents. CFA dispenses with the extraneous and the impractical and focuses on real-life street combat. Unlike so many martial arts, CFA is not about Zen, tournaments, or mixed martial arts competition. It doesn't teach or practice katas or rituals. CFA is about defending the sanctity of your space and body, and perhaps your life!

CFA draws upon the concepts of numerous modern sciences and disciplines, including police and military science, criminal justice, criminology, sociology, human psychology, philosophy, histrionics, ballistics, physics, kinesics, proxemics, kinesiology, physiognomy, emergency medicine, crisis management, and human anatomy. As a result, it is a complete system of combat that can be adapted to the rigors of real world self-defense.

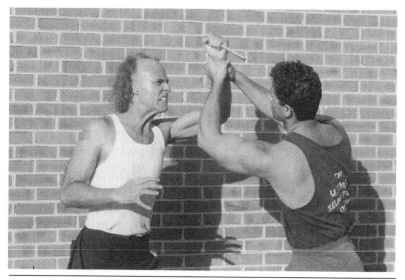

CFA is about teaching people how to really fight! In this photo, Sammy Franco (on the right) protects himself from a knife attack.

CONTEMPORARY FIGHTING ARTS - THE NAME SAYS IT ALL!

Before discussing the specific elements that make up CFA, it is important to explain how CFA obtained its unique name.

The first word, *Contemporary*, was selected because it refers to the system's modern, up-to-date orientation. Unlike traditional martial arts, CFA is specifically designed to meet the challenges of our modern world.

The second term, *Fighting*, was chosen because it accurately describes CFA's combat orientation. After all, why not just call it Contemporary Martial Arts? There are two reasons for this. First, the word *martial* conjures up images of traditional and impractical martial art forms that are antithetical to the system. Second, why dilute a perfectly functional name when the word *fighting* defines the system so succinctly? After all, Contemporary Fighting Arts is about teaching people how to really fight.

Let's look at the last word, *Arts*. In the subjective sense, the word *art* refers to the combat skills that are acquired through arduous study, practice, and observation. The bottom line is that effective street-fighting skills will require consistent practice and attention. For example, something as seemingly basic as an elbow strike will actually require hundreds of hours of practice to perfect.

The pluralization of art reflects CFA's protean instruction. The various components of CFA's training (e.g., firearms training, stick fighting, ground fighting, natural body weapon mastery) have all truly earned their status as individual art forms and, as such, require years of consistent study and practice to perfect.

To acquire a greater understanding of CFA, here is a brief overview of the system's three vital components: the physical, mental, and spiritual.

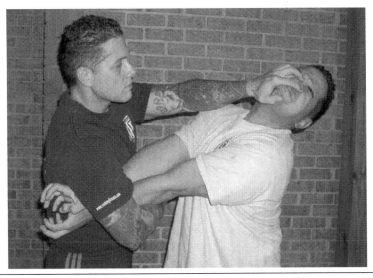

Contemporary Fighting Arts (CFA) is more than a self defense system, its a one-of-a-kind martial arts style geared for real world self defense.

PHYSICAL COMPONENT

The physical component of CFA focuses on the physical development of a fighter, including combat conditioning, weapon and technique mastery, and combat attributes.

Combat Conditioning

If you are going to prevail in a street fight, you must be physically fit. It's that simple. In fact, you will never master the tools and skills of combat unless you're in excellent physical shape. In CFA, combat conditioning comprises the following three broad components: cardiorespiratory conditioning, muscular-skeletal conditioning, and proper body composition.

Weapon and Technique Mastery

In CFA, we teach students both armed and unarmed methods of combat. Unarmed fighting requires that you master a complete arsenal of natural body weapons and techniques.

Students also receive instruction in specific methods of armed fighting. CFA's weapons program consists of natural body weapons, firearms, knives and edged weapons, kubotans, single and double sticks, makeshift weaponry, the side-handle baton (for law enforcement only), and oleoresin capsicum (OC), or pepper spray.

Combat Attributes

CFA also has a wide variety of training drills and methodologies designed to develop and sharpen combat attributes, which are specific qualities that enhance a fighter's combat skills. Included in these are power, speed, accuracy, timing, and balance.

We use more than 200 unique training methodologies in CFA. Each one is scientifically designed to prepare students for the hard-core realities of combat. There are also three specific training methodologies used to develop and sharpen the fundamental attributes and skills of armed and unarmed fighting, including proficiency training, conditioning training, and street training.

MENTAL COMPONENT

The mental component focuses on the cerebral aspects of a fighter, including the development of the killer instinct, strategic/tactical awareness, analysis/ integration skills, philosophy, and cognitive skills.

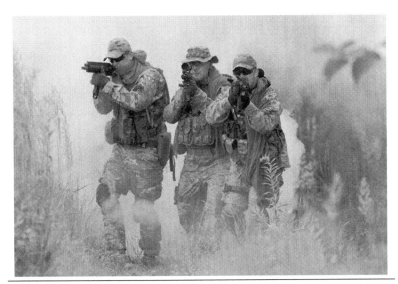

Contemporary Fighting Arts has a several unique military combat training programs. Our mission is to provide today's modern soldier with the knowledge, skills and attitude necessary to survive a wide variety of real world combat scenarios.

Killer Instinct

The killer instinct is a vicious combat mentality that surges to your consciousness and turns you into a fierce fighter free of fear, anger, and apprehension. In CFA we strive to tap the killer instinct in everyone. Visualization and crisis rehearsal are just two techniques we use to develop, refine, and channel this extraordinary source of strength and energy so that it can be used to its full potential.

Strategic/Tactical Awareness

In CFA, there are three unique categories of strategic awareness that will diminish the likelihood of losing a fight. They are criminal awareness, situational awareness, and self-awareness. When developed, these essential skills prepare you to assess a wide variety of threats instantaneously and accurately.

CFA also teaches students to assess a variety of other critical factors, including the assailant's demeanor, intent, range, and positioning and weapon capability, as well as such environmental issues as escape routes, barriers, terrain, and makeshift weaponry.

Analysis and Integration Skills

CFA's most advanced practitioners have sound insight and understanding of a wide range of sciences and disciplines. They include human anatomy, kinesiology, criminal justice, sociology, kinesics, proxemics, combat physics, emergency medicine, crisis management, histrionics, police and military science, the psychology of aggression, and the role of archetypes.

Philosophy

Philosophical resolution is essential to a fighter's mental confidence and clarity. Anyone learning the art of war must find the ultimate answers to questions concerning the use of violence in defense of himself or others.

Cognitive Skills

Cognitive exercises are also important for improving one's fighting skills. CFA uses visualization and crisis rehearsal scenarios to improve general body mechanics, tools and techniques, and maneuvers, as well as tactic selection. Mental clarity, concentration, and emotional control are also developed to enhance one's ability to call upon the controlled killer instinct.

SPIRITUAL COMPONENT

In CFA, the spiritual component is acquired slowly and progressively. During the challenging quest of combat training, one begins to tap the higher qualities of human nature, those elements of our being that inherently enable us to know right from wrong and good from evil. As we slowly develop this aspect of our total self, we begin to strengthen qualities profoundly important to the "truth." Such qualities are essential to growth through the mastery of inner peace, the clarity of "vision," and recognition of universal truths.

CHAPTER 1

THE FIRST-STRIKE PRINCIPLE

first strike *n*: The initial use of strategic nuclear weapons against a nuclear-armed adversary, theorized as feasible only if the attacker can destroy the adversary's retaliatory capacity.

—The American Heritage Dictionary
1993

THE FIRST STRIKE

Whenever you are threatened by a dangerous adversary and there is no way to escape safely, you must strike first, strike fast, strike with authority, and keep the pressure on. This offensive strategy is known as the first-strike principle, and it's essential to the process of neutralizing a formidable adversary in a self-defense altercation.

Basically, a first strike is defined as the strategic application of proactive force designed to interrupt the initial stages of an assault before it becomes a self-defense situation.

One inescapable fact about street self-defense is that the longer the fight lasts, the greater your chances of serious injury or even death. Common sense suggests that you must end the fight as quickly as possible. Striking first is the best method of achieving this tactical objective because it permits you to neutralize your assailant swiftly while, at the same time, precluding his ability to retaliate effectively. No time is wasted, and no unnecessary risks are taken.

When it comes to reality based self-defense, the element of surprise is invaluable. Launching the first strike gives you the upper hand because it allows you to hit the criminal adversary suddenly and unexpectedly. As a result, you demolish his defenses and ultimately take him out of the fight.

DON'T GET CONFUSED

Don't confuse the first-strike principle with the single-attack methodology. The single attack (or simple attack) is one of the five conventional methods of fighting whereby the fighter delivers a solitary offensive strike, or it may involve a series of discrete probes or one swift and powerful strike aimed at terminating the fight. Whatever the strategy, the single attack is clearly unsuitable for street self-defense.

First, in a volatile street confrontation, what sense does it make to remain uncommitted to the fight? I can assure you that you cannot neutralize an opponent by lingering at the perimeter of the encounter. Rather than toying around with single probes like jabbing punches and other "feelers," you must commit yourself 100 percent with the most effective flurry of blows appropriate to the ranges, angles, and use of force justification that present themselves.

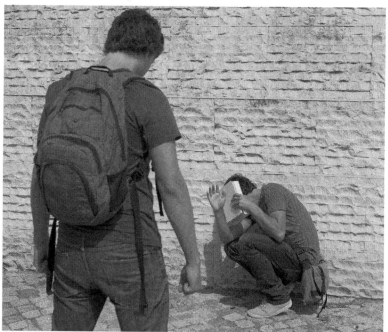

Remember in your younger days when a schoolyard fight was over after the first punch was thrown? Little did you know that you were employing the first-strike principle.

WARNING! AVOID BEING A DEFENSIVE FIGHTER

A defensive fighter is one who permits his adversary to seize and maintain offensive control in a fight. Beware! This defensive mind-set can get you killed in street combat. Simply put, allowing your antagonist the opportunity to deliver the first strike is tactical suicide. It's like allowing a gunslinger to draw his pistol first.

Never forget that in unarmed combat, if you permit the adversary to strike first, he might injure or possibly kill you, and he will most certainly force you into an irreversible defensive flow that can preclude you from issuing an effective counterattack.

Second, you cannot afford to gamble that one perfectly executed kick, punch, or strike will end the fight. Don't get me wrong - it's not that it can't be accomplished. I know for a fact that a powerful and accurately placed blow can end a fight. However, single-strike victories are few and far between.

The first-strike principle, however, is much different from the single attack because it's a constituent of your overall compound attack. It is not predicated on one isolated strike. Your preemptive strike is just one of the many offensive blows that shower your opponent.

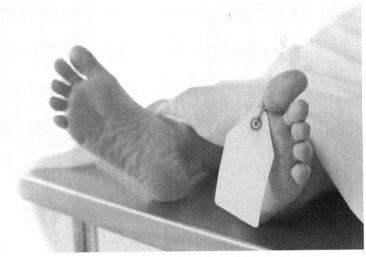

A defensive fighter can be found in one of two places: the hospital or the cemetery.

Employing the first-strike principle requires an offensive mentality that *compels you to act rather than react*. You must be aggressive and take affirmative and absolute control of the situation by making all the decisions and acting immediately without apprehension or trepidation.

Unfortunately, most martial art instructors teach their students to wait for their opponent to make the first move. *Big mistake!* In the mean streets, this reactive type of approach will get you a one-way trip to the city morgue.

There are also self-defense practitioners who are simply too timid to take the initiative and hit first. Many won't strike first because they simply don't know how to execute a preemptive strike successfully. Others are uncertain about the legal requirements and justifications, and, as a result, they second-guess their instincts, hesitate, and end up kissing the pavement. Therefore, it's imperative that you have a basic understanding of the legal requirements of launching a preemptive strike in a self-defense situation.

IT IS FAR BETTER

In all forms of combat it is far better for you to

- Act rather than react
- Lead rather than follow
- Attack rather than defend
- Strike rather than block
- Be decisive rather than indecisive

FIRST-STRIKE JUSTIFICATIONS

The most difficult aspect of the first-strike principle is determining *exactly when a person can strike first*. Well, because every self-defense situation is going to be different, there is no simple answer. However, there are some fundamental elements that must be present if you are going to launch a preemptive strike.

First, you must never use force against another person unless it is absolutely justified. Force is broken down into two levels: lethal and nonlethal. Lethal force is defined as the amount of force that can cause serious bodily injury or death. Nonlethal force is an amount of force that does not cause serious bodily injury or death.

Keep in mind that any time you use physical force against another person, you run the risk of having a civil suit filed against you. Anyone can hire a lawyer and file a suit for damages. Likewise, anyone can file a criminal complaint against you. Whether criminal charges will be brought against you depends upon the

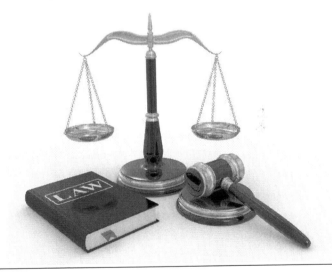

There is an interesting paradox facing all self-defense and martial art experts: the more highly trained in combat tactics, the higher the standard of care you must observe when protecting yourself and others.

prosecutor's or grand jury's view of the facts. Nevertheless, I can tell you that if you are trained in the martial arts, you will be held to a much higher standard of behavior by a jury of your peers.

Second, the first-strike principle should only be used as an act of protection against unlawful injury or the immediate risk of unlawful injury. If you decide to launch a preemptive strike against your adversary, you'd better be certain that a reasonable threat exists and that it is absolutely necessary to protect yourself from immediate danger.

Please remember, the decision to launch a preemptive strike must always be a last resort, after all other means of avoiding violence have been exhausted.

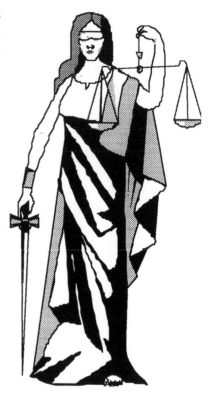

The first-strike principle is a particularly troublesome angle to self-defense and legal liability. Always be certain that your offensive actions are warranted and justified in the eyes of the law.

DOES A REASONABLE THREAT EXIST?

To determine whether a reasonable threat exists, you must assess your situation accurately. Assessment is the process of rapidly gathering and analyzing information and then accurately evaluating it in terms of threat and danger. In general, there are two factors to assess prior to launching a first strike: the environment and the adversary. Let's start with the environment and its related elements.

THE ENVIRONMENT

Because a criminal attack can occur anywhere, you must quickly evaluate the strategic implications of your environment, which is made up of your immediate surroundings, such as a street corner, parking lot, football stadium, golf course, grocery store, gas station, or the beach.

There are six essential factors to consider when assessing your environment: escape routes, barriers, makeshift weapons, terrain, positions of cover, and positions of concealment. Let's take a look at each one.

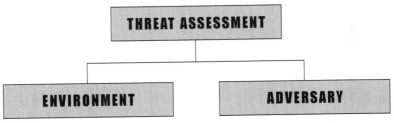

When determining whether a reasonable threat exists, you must assess the environment and the adversary.

Escape Routes

These are the various avenues or exits that allow you to flee from the threatening situation safely. Some possible escape routes are windows, fire escapes, doors, gates, escalators, fences, walls, bridges, and staircases.

Barriers

A barrier is any object that obstructs the assailant's path of attack. At the very least, barriers give you some distance and some time, and they may give you some safety - at least temporarily. A barrier, however, must have the structural integrity to perform the particular function that you have assigned it. Barriers are everywhere and include such things as large desks, doors, automobiles, Dumpsters, large trees, fences, walls, heavy machinery, and large vending machines.

Makeshift Weapons

These are common, everyday objects that can be converted into hand-held self-defense weapons. As with a barrier, a makeshift weapon must be appropriate to the function you have assigned to it. You won't be able to knock your adversary out with a car antenna, but you could whip it across his eyes and temporarily blind him. You could knock your assailant unconscious with a good, heavy flashlight, but you could not use it to shield yourself from a knife attack. Makeshift weapons can be broken down into the following four types: striking, distracting, shielding, and cutting.

Terrain

This is a critical environmental factor. What are the strategic implications of the terrain on which you are standing? Will the surface area interfere with your ability to fight your adversary? Terrain falls into one of these two possible categories:

- **Stable** (principally characterized as stationary, compact, dense, hard, flat, dry, or solid ground)
- **Unstable** (principally characterized as mobile, uneven, flexible, slippery, wet, or rocky ground).

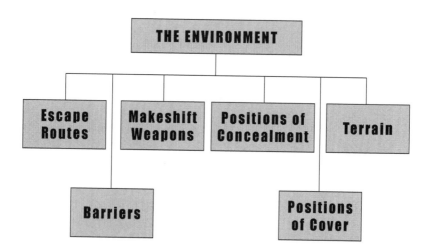

Positions of Cover

A position of cover is any object or location that temporarily protects you from an assailant's gunfire. Some examples include large concrete utility poles, large rocks, thick trees, an engine block, the corner of a building, concrete steps, and so on. Positions of cover are important not only because they protect you from gunfire but because they buy you some time and allow you to assess the situation from a position of safety. When choosing a position of cover, avoid selecting the following objects because bullets can penetrate them:

- internal doors
- small trees
- car doors
- all glass windows
- dry wall
- tall grass
- car trunks
- overturned tables
- trash cans
- shrubbery
- fences

Positions of Concealment

These are various locations or objects that allow you to hide from your adversary temporarily. Positions of concealment are most commonly used to evade engagement with your assailant(s), and they permit you to attack with the element of surprise. Positions of concealment include trees, shrubbery, doors, the dark, walls, stairwells, cars, and other large and tall objects.

WARNING: *Don't forget that positions of concealment will not protect you from an assailant's gunfire.*

THE ADVERSARY

Prior to launching your first strike, you must assess the source of danger. Who is posing the reasonable threat? Is it someone you know, or is it a complete stranger? Is it one guy or two or more? What are his intentions in confronting you? Pay very close attention to all available clues, especially nonverbal indicators. Your answers to these important questions will shape your overall tactical response. There are five essential factors to consider when assessing a threatening adversary prior to a self-defense situation: demeanor, intent, range, positioning, and weapon capability.

Demeanor

What is the adversary's outward behavior? Watch for both verbal and nonverbal clues. For example, is he shaking, or is he calm and collected? Are his shoulders hunched or relaxed? Are his hands clenched? Is his neck taut? Is he clenching his teeth? Is he breathing hard? Does he seem angry, frustrated, or confused? Does he seem high on drugs? Is he mentally ill or simply intoxicated? What is he saying? How is he saying it? Is he making sense? Is his speech slurred? What is his tone of voice? Is he talking rapidly or methodically? Is he cursing and angry?

Remember that all of these verbal and nonverbal cues are essential in accurately assessing the assailant's overall demeanor and adjusting your tactical response accordingly.

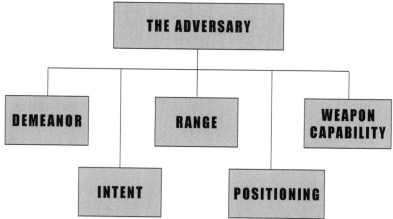

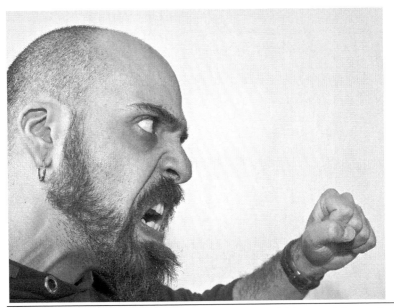

Remember, both verbal and nonverbal cues are essential in accurately assessing the assailant's overall demeanor and adjusting your tactical response accordingly.

CAN YOU RECOGNIZE THE THREAT OF VIOLENCE?

Many physical attacks are prefaced by various signs of aggression. What follow are some nonverbal cues of possible violence:

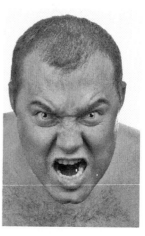

- Red face
- Heavy breathing
- Veins protruding from face or neck.
- Clenched teeth or fists
- Taut neck
- Sweating
- Hunched shoulders
- Shoulder shifts
- Target stares (e.g., looks at jaw, groin)
- Adversary's looks through you (the "1,000-yard stare")
- Hand concealment
- Parental finger (pointing finger in chest or face)
- Pacing back and forth or rapid forward movement

Here are a few verbal cues that violence is probable:

- Excessive swearing
- Screaming and yelling
- Threats or challenges
- Incoherent speech

Intent

Once you have assessed the adversary's demeanor, you're in a much better position to assess his intent. In other words, why is this person confronting you? Does he intend to rob or kill you? Is he trying to harass you? Is he seeking vengeance for something you have done? Or is he a troublemaker looking to pick a fight with you? Determining the assailant's intent is perhaps the most important assessment factor, but it also can be the most difficult.

Range

Range is the spatial relationship between you and your adversary. In unarmed combat, for example, there are three possible ranges from which your adversary can launch his attack: kicking, punching, and grappling. When assessing your adversary, you'll need to recognize the strategic implications and advantages of his range immediately. For example, is he close enough to land a punch effectively? Is he at a distance from which he could kick you? Is he in a range that would allow him to grab hold of you and take you down to the ground? Is he within range to slash you with a knife or strike you with a bludgeon? Is the assailant moving closer to you? If so, how fast? Does the assailant continue to move forward when you step back?

Positioning

This is the spatial relationship between you and the adversary in terms of threat, tactical escape, and target selection. In street combat, it's important to understand the strategic implications of the assailant's positioning before and during the fight. For example, is he standing squarely or sideways? Is he mounted on top of you in a ground fight? Or is he inside your leg guard? What anatomical targets does the adversary present you with? Is he blocking a door or any other escape route? Is his back to a light source? Is he close to your only possible makeshift weapon? Are multiple assailants closing in on you? Is he firing his gun from a position of cover or concealment?

Weapon Capability

Always try to determine whether your adversary is armed or unarmed. If he is carrying a weapon, what type is it? Does he have an effective delivery method for the particular weapon? Is he armed with more than one weapon? If so, where are they located? There are four general points of concern when assessing the assailant's weapon capability: hand/fingers, general behavior, clothing, and location.

Hands/Fingers

When strategically scanning your adversary for weapons, quickly glance at his hands and all his fingertips. Can you see them? Is one hand behind him or in his pockets? If you cannot see his fingers, he could be palming a knife or some other edged weapon. Remember to be extremely cautious when the assailant's arms are crossed in front of his body or when he keeps his hands in his pockets.

General Behavior

How is the assailant behaving? For example, does he pat his chest frequently (as a weapon security check)? Does he act apprehensive, nervous, or uneasy? Or does he seem to be reaching for something? Is your assailant's body language inconsistent with his verbal statements?

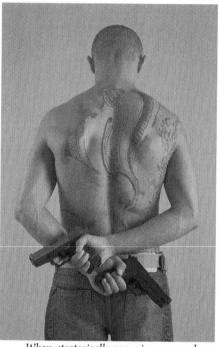

When strategically scanning your adversary for weapons, quickly glance at his hands and all his fingertips. If you can't see both of his hands, he could be concealing a weapon.

Clothing

What the assailant is wearing can also clue you in on what he may be concealing. For example, is the assailant wearing a knife sheath on his belt? Could there be a knife concealed in his boot? At other times you may have to be a bit more analytical. For example, is your assailant wearing a jacket when it is too hot for one? Could it be to conceal a gun or edged weapon at his waist or shoulder?

Location

Does the assailant seem suspiciously rooted to a particular spot? Or is he running back to his car, possibly to get his gun? Is he close enough to grab that beer bottle on the bar? How far is the assailant from a makeshift weapon?

DON'T STEREOTYPE YOUR ADVERSARY

It's important to consider that the person you must strike first may not fit your stereotype of a dangerous adversary. I know of several people, for example, who erroneously imagine that they will be confronted by a "typical scumbag"—a loathsome, contemptuous male of another race. But what if your adversary turns out to be a clean-cut business executive of your own ethnic background who menacingly waves his fist in your face? Will you be able launch a first strike without trepidation? I hope so—for your sake.

RESOLVE MORAL ISSUES NOW

Before you move on to Chapter 2, it's very important that you raise and resolve moral issues concerning the use of a first strike in defense of yourself and others. Do your religious or philosophical beliefs permit you to launch a preemptive strike? Could you take the life of another in defense of yourself or a loved one?

Ironically, your biggest enemy in a combat situation is often your mixed-up moral conscience. For some people, being forced to execute a first strike can create apprehension during the encounter. This is because of incorrect perceptions or misinterpretation of many religious or associated beliefs.

DECISIONS, DECISIONS, DECISIONS

Mental decisiveness can significantly minimize danger and risk. The more decisions you're able to make before an encounter with an opponent, the better off you will be. Basically, there are three types of decisions that must be addressed if you expect to launch a successful first strike:

Moral • Legal • Tactical

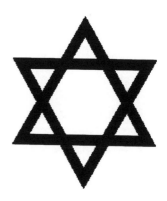

Your biggest enemy prior to launching a first strike is often your mixed-up moral conscience. This is because of incorrect perceptions or misinterpretations of many religious or associated beliefs.

Our culture and system of government are both based on the Judeo-Christian ethic. With this in mind, our parents, teachers, friends, etc., have ingrained morality issues in us. Therefore, such common statements as "turn the other cheek," "pick on someone your own size," or "don't hit a woman," often leave you with the fatal perception that a smaller or female adversary should be treated differently, when, in reality, anyone—regardless of size, age, gender, race, or appearance—has the potential to destroy you.

The Bible can also be easily misinterpreted regarding the use of deadly force. For example, the commandment "Thou shalt not kill" can cause people to hesitate to employ lethal techniques. A more accurate translation of this commandment is, "Thou shalt not murder" (Exodus 20:13; murder being the unjustifiable taking of another human life). Some people feel they have no right to kill another human being.

When using deadly force, your objective is not to take life from another human being, but to stop your enemy from causing you grievous bodily harm or possible death. However, the possibility of the enemy dying should be of no consequence to you. The bottom line is, when warranted and justified, killing another person is permitted even under God's law.

As a law-abiding citizen, you clearly have the right by law to defend yourself under certain circumstances. Can you accept that, or does the possibility of a justified first strike induce moral doubts in your mind? If you have any apprehension or your conscience precludes you from initiating a preemptive strike, then do not attempt to execute any of the principles and techniques discussed in this book! Let me remind you that executing a first strike requires a particular type of psychological and emotional makeup—it's not for everyone!

YOU CAN DO IT!

At this point I am sure you realize that successfully delivering a first strike is not such an easy task. However, the information is accessible to anyone with the sincere desire to learn and the willingness to put forth the effort. The techniques and procedures outlined in this book will equip you with the necessary knowledge, skills, and attitude to do the job right. When training, remember this simple equation:

Knowledge + Skills + Attitude = Street Survival

BEWARE: *The self-defense techniques and principles contained herein are dangerous. Be ever mindful that you are personally and socially responsible for this knowledge and power.*

WHAT'S NEXT?

There are several prerequisites that you must possess if you are to successfully employ the first-strike principle in a fight. These are identified and discussed in detail in Chapter 2.

FIRST STRIKE

FIRST-STRIKE PREREQUISITES

"Why take by force what you could obtain through deception?"

—Sammy Franco

Before you can successfully employ the first-strike principle in a street fight, there are 11 prerequisites that you must understand and master: range proficiency, stances, mobility, body weapon mastery, target awareness, combat attributes, compound attack and offensive flow, the "Gemini" principle, the fifth-column tactic, fear management, and killer instinct.

RANGE PROFICIENCY

A street fight is unfair and unpredictable. It can occur anytime and anywhere. If you want to successfully launch a first strike (or be victorious in a fight), then you'd better be range proficient. Range proficiency is the skill and ability to fight your adversary in all three distances of unarmed combat (kicking range, punching range, and grappling range).

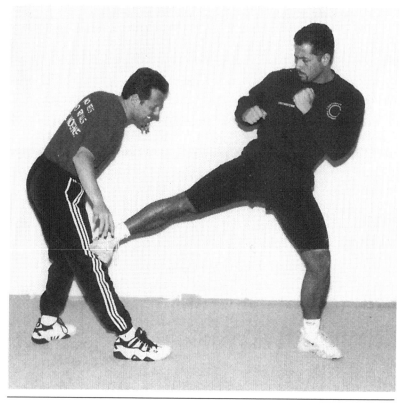

The kicking range of unarmed combat.

Kicking Range

The farthest distance of unarmed combat is kicking range. At this distance you are usually too far away to strike with your hands, so you use your legs to strike your opponent. Kicking techniques are safe, economical, and powerful, and they include vertical, push, side, and hook kicks.

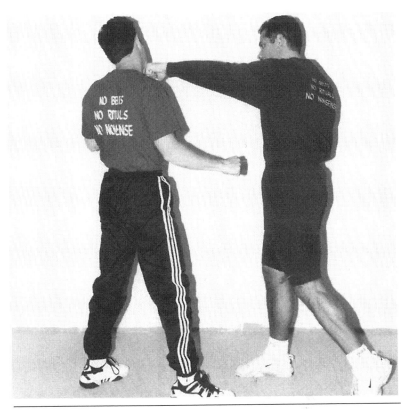

The punching range of unarmed combat.

Punching Range

Punching range is the midrange of unarmed fighting. At this distance, you are close enough to the enemy to strike him with your hands and fists. Punching-range techniques are quick, efficient, and effective, and they include finger jabs, palm heels, lead straights, rear crosses, hooks, uppercuts, web-hand strikes, and hammer fists.

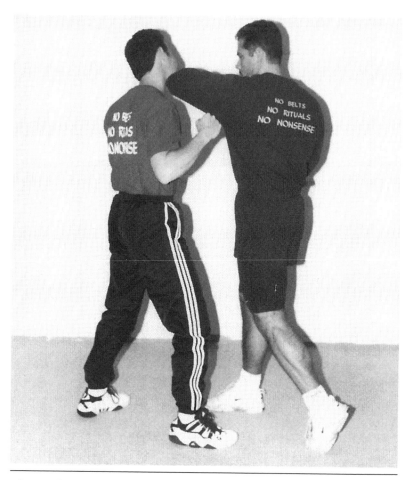

The grappling range (vertical plane) of unarmed combat.

Grappling Range

The third and closest range of unarmed combat is grappling range. At this distance, you are too close to your opponent to kick or execute some hand strikes, so you would use close-quarter tools and techniques to neutralize your adversary.

Grappling range is divided into two different planes: vertical and horizontal. In the vertical plane, you would deliver impact techniques,

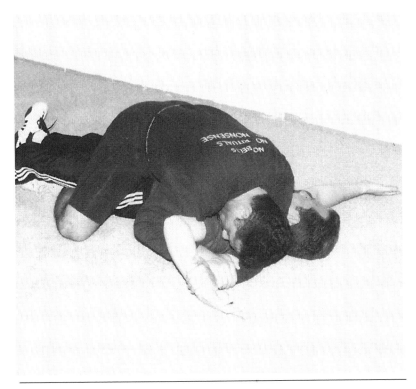

The grappling range (horizontal plane) of unarmed combat.

some of which include elbow and knee strikes, head butts, gouging and crushing tactics, and biting and tearing techniques.

In the horizontal plane, you are ground fighting with your enemy and can deliver all of the previously mentioned techniques, including various submission holds, locks, and chokes.

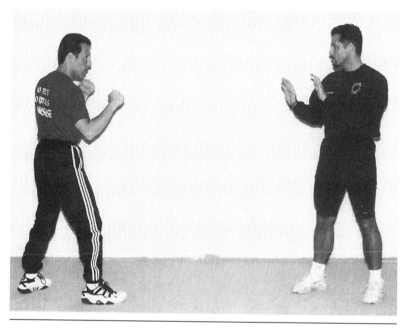

The neutral zone of unarmed combat.

DON'T FORGET THE NEUTRAL ZONE

In unarmed combat, the neutral zone is *not* a range of combat engagement. It is the distance at which neither you nor your opponent can physically strike one another. Although the neutral zone is the ideal place to be when assessing your environment and your adversary, it's the wrong place to be when attempting to launch a first strike.

NOTE: *To initiate a preemptive strike effectively, you must be standing in one of the three combat ranges, preferably the punching or grappling range.*

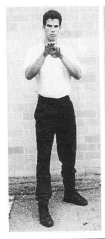 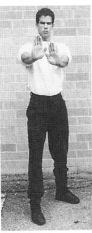 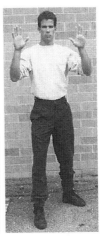 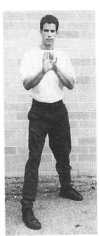

When assuming the first-strike stance, avoid pointing your fingertips at the adversary. It looks too threatening.

Extending your arms out to the enemy is another common mistake with the first-strike stance. You will be unable to launch an attack.

When assuming the grappling-range first-strike stance, don't let your arms spread out too far apart. You will be opening yourself to a wide range of possible attacks.

Foot positioning is another important aspect. Don't lock your knees or let your feet spread too far apart. It looks too aggressive, and you'll inhibit your mobility.

STANCES

A stance defines your ability to launch a first strike, and it plays a material role in the outcome of a fight. There are two stances that need to be developed: first strike and fighting. Let's begin with the first-strike stance.

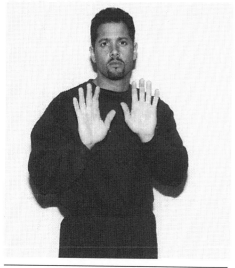

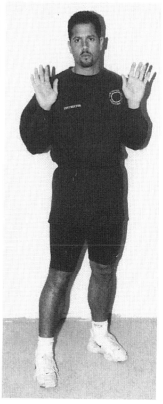

Your eyes are not misleading you, the first-strike stance is practically identical to the de-escalation stance. Did you know that the only difference between CFA's de-escalation stance and the first-strike stance is the intent?

First-Strike Stance

The first-strike stance is used *prior* to initiating your first strike. It facilitates "invisible deployment" of a preemptive strike while simultaneously protecting your vital targets against various possible counterattacks.

When assuming the first-strike stance, have both of your feet approximately shoulder width apart, knees slightly bent with your body weight evenly distributed over each leg. Blade your body at a 45-degree angle from your adversary. This position will help situate your centerline at a protective angle from your opponent, enhance your balance, promote mobility, and set up your first-strike weapons. Next, make certain to keep your torso, pelvis, head, and back straight.

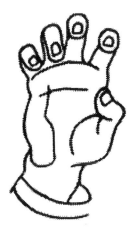

One of the most common mistakes made with the first-srike stance is the tendency to curl your finger inward. This type of clawing configuration looks aggressive and threatening, which defeats the purpose of your stance.

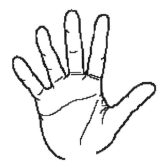

Another common mistake is to fan your fingers out. This hand articulation indicates alarm or fright to the adversary.

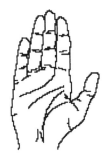 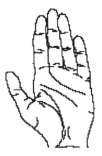

Here is an example of the correct way to hold your hands. Notice that both of your hands are open, relaxed, and up to protect the upper gates of your centerline.

TENSION AND RANGE

I would be remiss if I didn't mention that there is a direct correlation between ranges of engagement and physiological stress. Generally speaking, in unarmed combat, the closer you are to your opponent, the greater physiological tension you will experience. The only sure-fire method of relaxing in close proximity to your adversary is to be psychologically and physically prepared for combat.

And always stay relaxed and ready. Do not make the mistake of tensing your neck, shoulders, arms, or thighs. This muscular tension will most certainly throw off your timing, retard the speed of your movements, and telegraph your intentions.

Your hand positioning is another critical component of the first-strike stance. When confronted with an opponent in the kicking and punching ranges of unarmed combat, keep both of your hands open, relaxed, and up to protect the upper gates of your centerline. Both of your palms should be facing the opponent with your lead arm bent between 90 and 120 degrees, while your rear arm should be approximately eight inches from your chin. When faced with an opponent in grappling range, keep both of your hands beside one another.

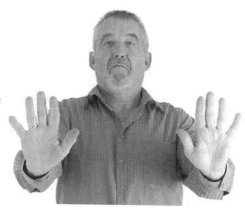

When employing the first strike stance, avoid extending your arms out to the adversary. This mistake will inhibit your ability to launch a first strike.

Fighting Stance

After you have successfully launched your first-strike weapon at your enemy, it's time to maintain a fighting stance. The fighting stance is a strategic and aggressive posture that facilitates maximum execution of your compound attack (aka, secondary strike weapons) while simultaneously protecting your anatomical targets.

When assuming the fighting stance, be certain to place your stronger and more coordinated side forward. For example, a right-handed person would stand with his right hand and foot facing his adversary. Next, blade your feet and body at a 45-degree angle from your assailant. This will keep your body targets back and away from direct strikes. Place your feet approximately shoulder width apart, with both knees slightly bent. Your legs will function like power springs to launch you through the ranges of unarmed combat. Try to maintain a 50 percent weight distribution. This will

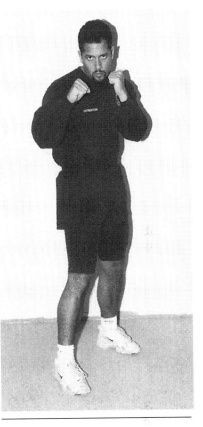

The fighting stance is the ideal vehicle for street combat; however, it should only be employed after you have launched your first-strike weapon.

provide you with the ability to move in any direction quickly and efficiently, as well as the necessary stability to defend against various strikes.

Your hand positioning is also critical. Keep both of your hands up. This will help protect your centerline and set up your body weapons. Your hands should be loosely fisted with your fingers curled and your wrists straight. This will prevent muscular tension and help increase the speed of your offensive and defensive movements. When holding your hand guard, make certain not to tighten your neck, shoulders, or arms. Finally, remember to keep your chin angled down. This reduces the likelihood of a knockout blow to the chin or a deadly strike to the windpipe.

MOBILITY

It is imperative that you remain mobile during the course of a fight. Mobility is critical because it makes it difficult for your opponent to hit you, while at the same time enhancing the power of your strikes.

Mobility is defined as your ability to move your body quickly and economically. This can be accomplished through basic footwork. The safest footwork involves quick, economical steps performed on the balls of your feet, while you remain relaxed and balanced.

Basic Footwork

Basic footwork can be used for both offensive and defensive purposes, and it is structured around four general directions: advancing, retreating, sidestepping right, and sidestepping left.

Moving Forward (Advancing)

From your fighting stance, first move your front foot forward (approximately 18 to 24 inches) and then move your rear foot an equal distance.

Moving Backward (Retreating)

From your fighting stance, first move your rear foot backward (approximately 18 to 24 inches) and then move your front foot an equal distance.

Moving Right (Sidestepping Right)

From a fighting stance, first move your right foot to the right (approximately 18 to 24 inches) and then move your left foot an equal distance.

Moving Left (Sidestepping Left)

From a fighting stance, first move your left foot to the left (approximately 18 to 24 inches) and then move your left foot an equal distance.

NOTE: Practice these four movements every day for 10 to 15 minutes in front of a full-length mirror until your footwork is quick, balanced, and natural.

Advanced Footwork

Once you have mastered basic footwork, you can incorporate strategic circling into your cache of techniques. Strategic circling is an advanced form of footwork where the fighter uses his lead leg as a pivot point. This advanced footwork can be used defensively to evade an overwhelming assault or offensively to strike the enemy from a strategic angle. Strategic circling can be performed from either a right or left stance.

Circling Right (from a Right Stance)

From a right lead stance, step six to eight inches to the right with your right foot, and then use your right leg as a pivot point and wheel your entire rear leg to the right until the correct stance and positioning are acquired. Remember to keep both of your hands up.

Circling Left (from a Left Stance)

From a left lead stance, step six to eight inches to the left with your left foot and then use your left leg as a pivot point and wheel your entire rear leg to the left until the correct stance and positioning are acquired.

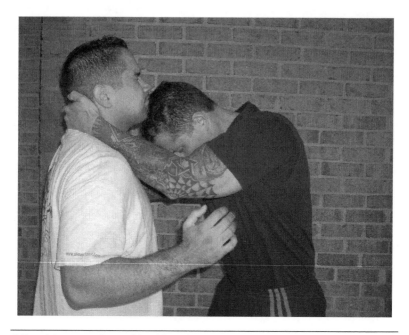

When delivering a forward head butt, be certain to make contact with the top portion of your forehead.

BODY WEAPON MASTERY

Your body is a lethal weapon! Actually, you have 14 natural body weapons that can be used in a fight. When properly developed, these tools have the capacity to disable, cripple, and even kill your adversary. *Keep in mind that the lethality of your body weapon is predicated on two important factors: the target that you select and the amount of force you deliver.* Having said that, let's take a look at each body weapon.

Head

When fighting in grappling range, your head can be used for butting your opponent's nose. Keep in mind that the head butt can be delivered in four different directions: forward, backward, right side, and left side.

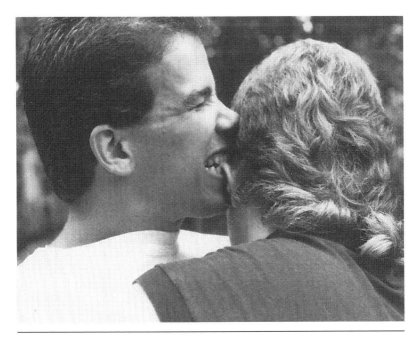

There is an important concern to biting in a street fight: you run the risk of contracting AIDS if your adversary is infected and you draw blood while biting him.

Teeth

The teeth can be used for biting anything on your opponent's body (e.g., nose, ears, throat, fingers). Remember to bite deeply into the assailant's flesh and shake your head vigorously.

Voice

Believe it or not, but your voice is also a weapon. When used correctly it can distract and shock your assailant, causing him to temporarily freeze. Yelling serves many purposes in combat. Yelling while fighting can distract, startle, and temporarily paralyze your enemy, allowing you a split-second advantage to deliver the first debilitating strike and thus gain offensive control. It can also be used to synchronize your state of mind with the physical process taking place.

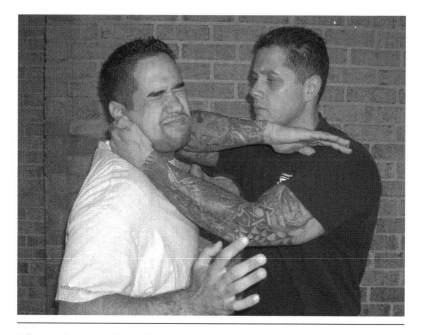

Elbow strikes are explosive, deceptive, and difficult to defend against.

Elbows

The elbows are devastating weapons that can generate tremendous power. Elbow strikes can be delivered vertically, diagonally, and horizontally to the opponent's nose, temple, chin, throat, solar plexus, and ribs.

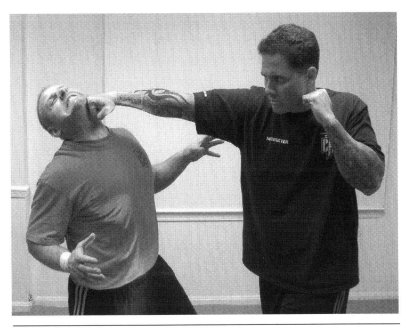

When landing your punch, remember to make contact with your center knuckle.

Fists/Knuckles

The fists are used for punching the opponent's temple, nose, chin, throat, solar plexus, ribs, and, in some cases, groin. Punching is an art form that requires considerable training and practice to master.

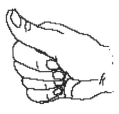 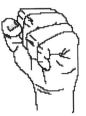

Left: One common mistake among novices is to punch with the fingers unclenched and the thumb extended. Right: The correct way to make a fist. Notice how the thumb is wrapped securely around the second and third knuckles.

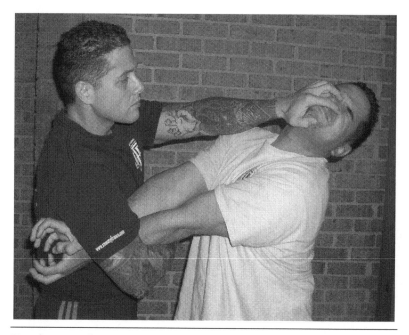

Your fingers can be an awesome weapon is a street fight. Make certain your actions are legally justified!

Fingers/Nails

Your fingers and nails can be used for jabbing, clawing, and gouging the opponent's eyes. They can also be used for pulling, tearing, and crushing his throat and testicles.

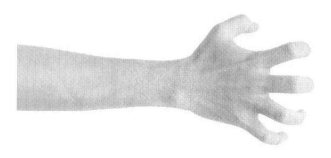

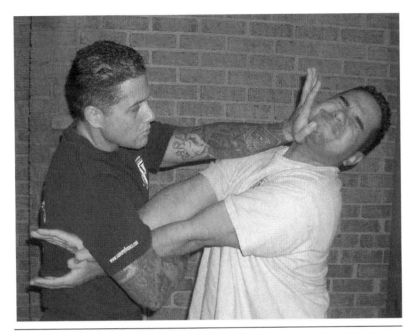

When striking with the heel of your palm, remember to torque your shoulders, hips, and foot into the direction of the blow.

Heel of the Palm

The heel of your palm can be used for delivering palm-heel strikes. A strike of the palm can be exceptionally powerful, and it is best delivered on a 45-degree angle to the opponent's nose or chin.

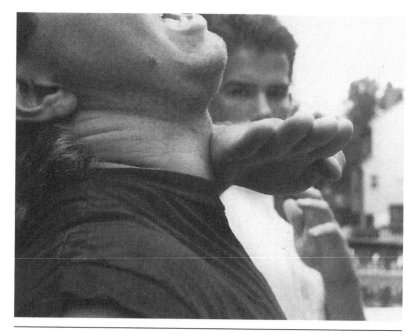

Beware! Striking with the edge of your hand can be lethal.

Edge of the Hand

The edge of your hand can be whipped horizontally into the opponent's nose or throat, causing severe injury or death. It can also be delivered vertically or diagonally to the back of his neck.

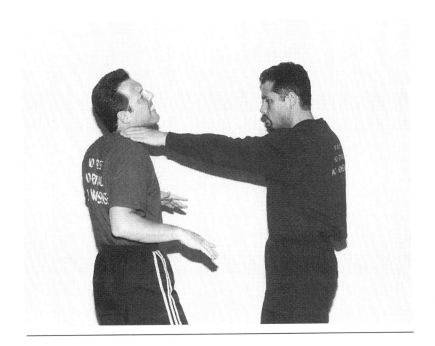

Web of the Hand

The web of your hand can be used to deliver web-hand strikes to the opponent's throat. When striking, be certain to keep your hand stiff with your palm facing down.

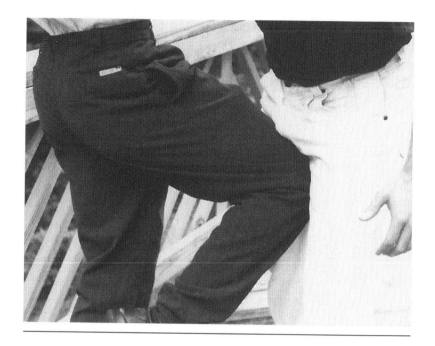

Knees

The knees are excellent grappling-range weapons that can bring down the most powerful of adversaries. Knee strikes can be delivered vertically and diagonally to the opponent's thigh, groin, ribs, solar plexus, and face.

OPEN-HAND OR FISTED STRIKES?

Are open-hand strikes (e.g., finger jabs, palm heels, web-hand strikes) or fisted blows (e.g., lead straight, rear cross, hook punches) the preferred weapons in a street fight? Although open-hand blows are generally safer to deliver than fisted strikes, both are essential for combat. Open-hand strikes are generally used as first-strike tools, and fisted blows constitute the majority of your secondary-strike arsenal.

Some people are reluctant to employ fisted strikes for fear that they will injure their hands. Be forewarned: When a fisted blow makes contact with the opponent's skull, it often results in a fractured hand. Therefore, it's essential that your fisted blow be delivered accurately and at the proper moment.

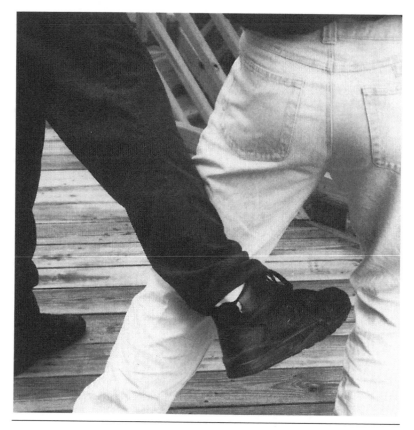

When kicking with your shinbone, always aim through your target.

Shins

The shinbone is another powerful body weapon that can quickly cripple an assailant. When striking with your shin, aim for the opponent's thigh or the side of his knees.

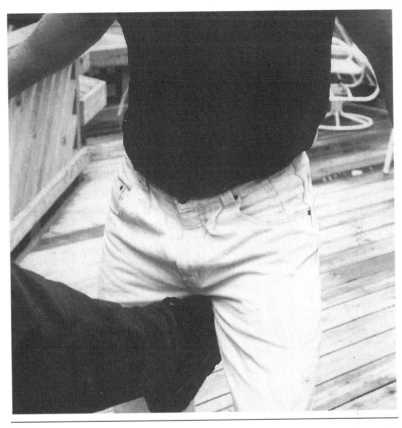

Kicking with your instep increases the power of your blow, prevents broken toes, and also lengthens the surface area of your strike.

Instep

The instep is used for delivering vertical kicks to the opponent's groin and, in some cases, his head.

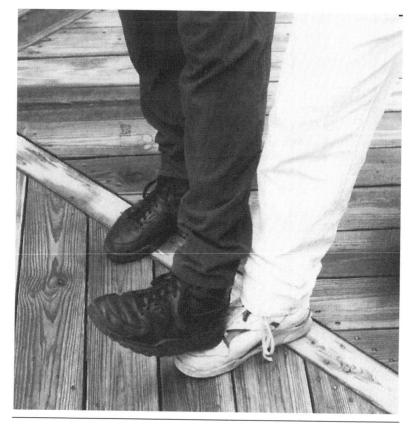

Never underestimate the effectiveness of a simple foot stomp.

Heel of the Foot

The heel of your foot is used for delivering side kicks to the opponent's thigh, knee, or shin. It can also be used to stomp on his toes.

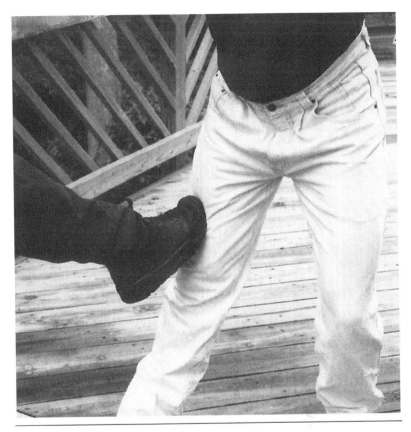

When striking with the ball of your foot, remember to pull your toes back to avoid jamming or breaking them.

Ball of the Foot

The ball of your foot is used for delivering push kicks to your opponent's thigh. It can also be used to deliver a quick snap kick into his shinbone.

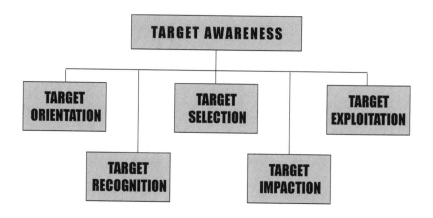

TARGET AWARENESS

The first-strike principle is useless unless you know exactly *where* and *when* to strike your adversary. In CFA, this is known as target awareness. Actually, target awareness is a culmination of five strategic principles: target orientation, target recognition, target selection, target impaction, and target exploitation. Following is a brief overview of each one.

Target Orientation

Target orientation means having a workable knowledge of the specific anatomical targets. Your opponent's anatomical targets are located in one of three possible target zones.

Zone 1 (Head Region)

Since this zone consists of targets related to the assailant's senses—including the eyes, temples, nose, chin, and back of neck—it will be your primary target for your first-strike weapons.

Zone 2 (Neck, Torso, Groin)

This zone consists of targets related to the assailant's breathing, including the throat, solar plexus, ribs, and testicles.

THE TARGET ZONES

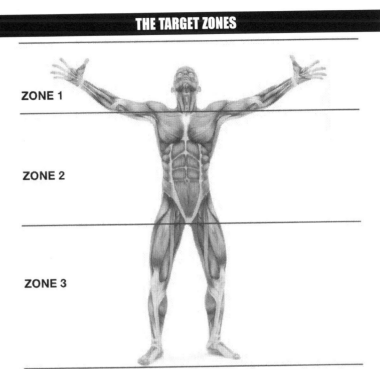

ZONE 1

ZONE 2

ZONE 3

Zone 3 (Legs and Feet)

This consists of anatomical targets related to the assailant's mobility, including the thighs, knees, shins, instep, and toes.

The illustration above will help acquaint you with these three targets.

Simply knowing the specific locations of various anatomical targets is not enough. Target orientation also requires that you have a strong understanding of the medical implications of striking these targets. As a matter of fact, every martial artist or combat specialist has the moral and legal responsibility to know the medical implications of every offensive strike and technique. A competent combatant must know exactly which anatomical targets will stun, incapacitate, disfigure, maim, or kill his adversary. Therefore, let's take a closer look at these targets and the medical implications of each.

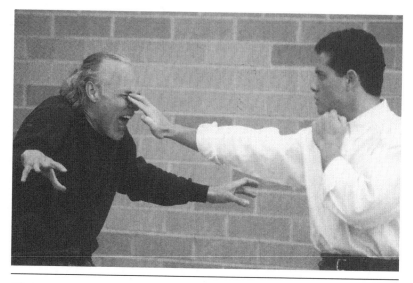

The eyes are extremely vulnerable.

Eyes: The eyes are ideal targets in street fighting because they are extremely sensitive and difficult to protect. The eyes can be poked, scratched, and gouged from a variety of angles and vantages. Depending on the force of your strike, attacking the eyes can cause numerous injuries, including watering of the eyes, hemorrhaging, blurred vision, temporary or permanent blindness, severe pain, rupture, shock, and even unconsciousness.

Temples: The temple or sphenoid bone is a thin, weak bone located on both sides of the skull approximately one inch from the assailant's eye. Because of its inherently weak structure and close proximity to the brain, a very powerful strike to this anatomical target can be deadly. Other possible injuries include unconsciousness, hemorrhaging, concussion, shock, and coma.

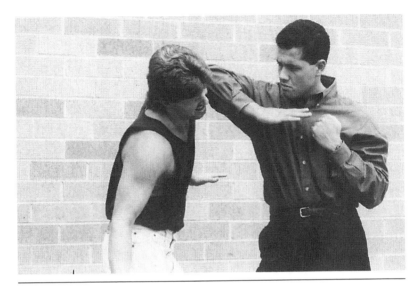

Beware: A powerful blow to the temple can be fatal.

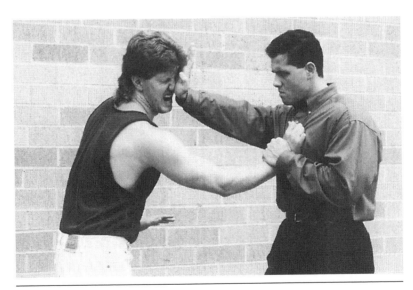

The nose is loaded with nerves and blood vessels. Here, the author attacks with a palm-heel strike.

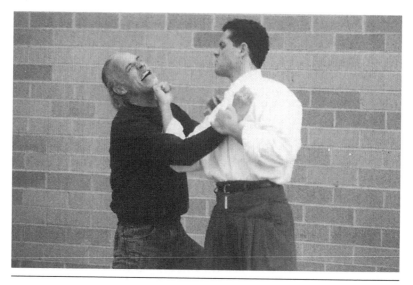

Sammy Franco strikes the opponent's "knockout button."

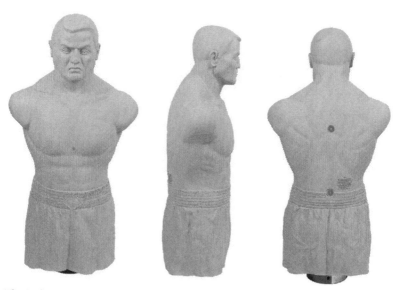

The Body Opponent Bag is one of the best training tools for developing target accuracy with all of your strikes.

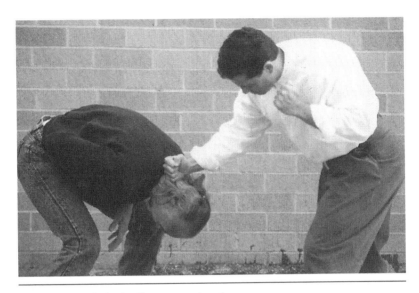

Franco attacks the back of his opponent's neck.

Nose: The nose is made up of a thin bone, cartilage, numerous blood vessels, and many nerves. It is a particularly good impact target because it stands out from the assailant's face and can be struck in three different directions (up, straight, down). A moderate blow can cause stunning pain, eye watering, temporary blindness, and hemorrhaging. A powerful strike can result in shock and unconsciousness.

Chin: The chin is also a good target for unarmed street combat. When the chin is struck at a 45-degree angle, shock waves are transmitted to the cerebellum and cerebral hemispheres of the brain, which could result in paralysis or immediate unconsciousness. Depending on the force of your blow, other possible injuries include broken jaw, concussion, and whiplash to the assailant's neck.

Back of Neck: The back of the assailant's neck consists of the first seven vertebrae of the spinal column, which enclose the spinal cord. The cord (and nerves) functions as a circuit board for nerve impulses from the brain to the body. The back of the neck is a lethal target

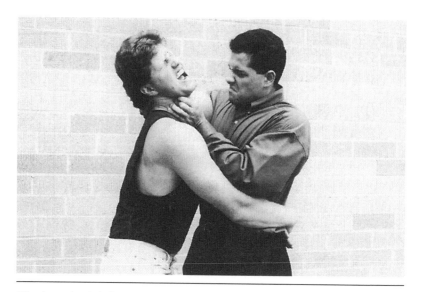

The throat is a lethal target. Be certain your actions are always justified.

because the vertebrae are poorly protected. A very powerful strike to the back of the assailant's neck can cause shock, unconsciousness, a broken neck, complete paralysis, coma, or death.

Throat: The throat is considered a lethal target because it is protected by only a thin layer of skin. This region consists of the thyroid, hyaline, cricoid cartilage, trachea, and larynx. The trachea, or windpipe, is a cartilaginous cylindrical tube that measures four and a half inches in length and approximately one inch in diameter. A direct and powerful strike to this target may result in unconsciousness, drowning by blood, massive hemorrhaging, strangulation, and death. If the thyroid cartilage is crushed, hemorrhaging will occur, the windpipe will quickly swell shut, and the assailant will die of suffocation.

Ribs: There are 12 pairs of ribs in the human body. Excluding the 11th and 12th ribs, the ribs are long, slender bones that are joined by the vertebral column in the back and the sternum and costal cartilage in the front. Since there are no 11th and 12th ribs (floating ribs) in the front, you

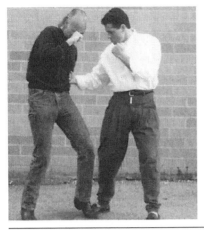

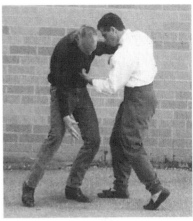

Sammy Franco strikes his opponent's ribs.

A powerful blow to the solar plexus can be devastating to your opponent.

should direct your strikes to the 9th and 10th ribs. A moderate strike to the anterior region of the ribs may cause severe pain and shortness of breath. An extremely powerful 45-degree blow could break one or more of the assailant's ribs and force it into a lung, resulting in the lung's collapse, internal hemorrhaging, air starvation, unconsciousness, excruciating pain, or death.

Solar Plexus: The solar plexus is a large collection of nerves situated below the sternum in the upper abdomen. A moderate blow to this area can cause nausea, pain, and shock, making it difficult for the adversary to breathe properly. A powerful strike to the solar plexus can result in severe abdominal pain and cramping, air starvation, or shock.

Groin: The testes can be kicked, punched, or crushed. A moderate kick or strike to an assailant's groin can cause a variety of possible reactions, including severe pain, nausea, vomiting, shortness of breath, or sterility. A powerful strike to the groin may crush the scrotum and the testes against the pubic bones, causing shock and unconsciousness.

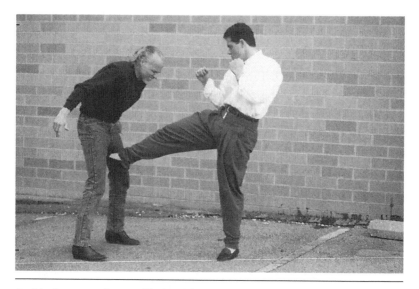

In this photo a quick vertical kick is delivered to the opponent's groin.

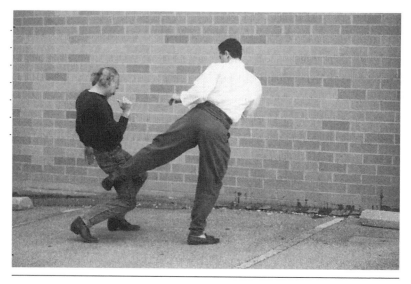

Many fighters overlook the thighs as a viable target in a street fight. The author delivers a powerful hook kick to his opponent's quadriceps.

Thighs: Because the thighs are large and difficult to protect, they make excellent striking targets in a fight. Although you can kick the thighs at a variety of different angles, the ideal location is the assailant's common peroneal nerve located on the side of the thigh, approximately four inches above the knee. Striking this area can result in extreme pain and immediate immobility of the afflicted leg. An extremely hard kick to the thigh may result in a fracture of the femur, internal bleeding, severe pain, intense cramping, and long-term immobility.

Knees: The knees are relatively weak joints that are held together by a number of supporting ligaments. When the assailant's leg is locked or fixed in position and a forceful strike is delivered to the front of the joint, the crucial ligaments will tear, resulting in excruciating pain, swelling, and immobility. Located on the front of the knee joint is the kneecap, or patella, which is made of a small, loose piece of bone. The patella is also vulnerable to possible dislocation by a direct, forceful kick. Severe pain, swelling, and immobility may also result.

Shins: The shins are also very sensitive targets because they are only protected by a thin layer of skin. A powerful kick delivered to this target may fracture it easily, resulting in extreme pain, hemorrhaging, and immobility of the afflicted leg.

Fingers: The fingers are exceptionally weak and vulnerable. They can easily be jammed, sprained, broken, torn, and bitten. Although a broken finger might not stop a determined fighter, it will certainly force him to release his hold. A broken finger will also make it very difficult for the assailant to clench his fist or hold a knife or bludgeon. When attempting to break the fingers, it's best to grab the finger securely and then forcefully tear backward against the knuckle.

Toes: In grappling range, a powerful stomp of your heel can break the small bones of the assailant's toes, causing severe pain and immediate immobility. Stomping on the assailant's toes is also one of the best ways for releasing many holds. Keep in mind that you should avoid attacking the toes if the attacker is wearing hard leather boots.

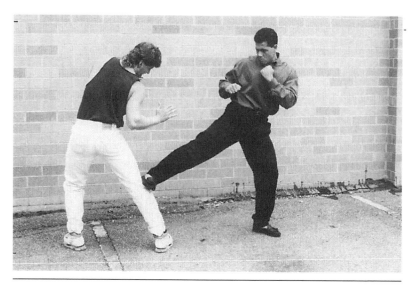

It is practically impossible to protect your knees from an attack. Here, Sammy Franco stops his opponent in his tracks with a side kick.

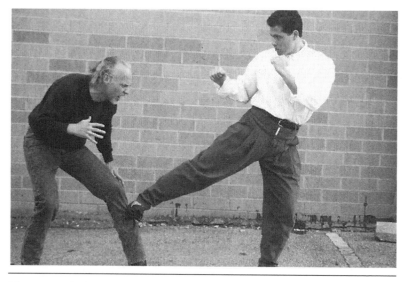

The opponent's shin is another effective target that can be attacked in a street fight.

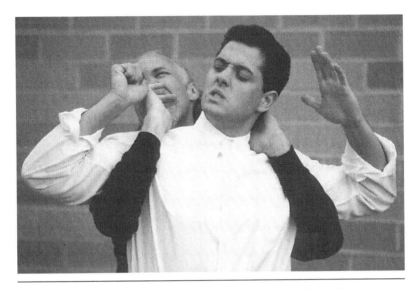

Tearing the opponent's fingers requires a vicious and determined attitude.

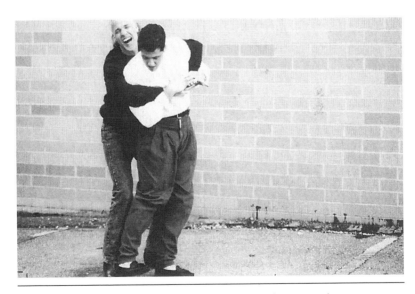

You can escape several grabs and holds by stomping on the opponent's toes.

ANTICIPATE THE HORROR

The vast majority of unarmed street fights occur at close range. This means that you will most likely hear your assailant's bones break... or hear him shriek in pain... or get some of his blood spattered on your hands or clothes. Unanticipated, such happenings can be extremely distracting during a street fight and can haunt your memories for a long time. However, if you anticipate the nitty-gritty residuals of unarmed combat, it is much less likely to be debilitating.

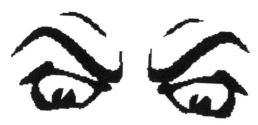

Eye-to-eye contact preceding a first strike is dangerous for a variety of logical reasons. The opponent's eyes will often provide no vital data, psych you out, draw your attention away from the immediate threat, or make you fall victim to a variety of visual feints.

Target Recognition

Target recognition is the ability to immediately recognize specific anatomical targets before or during a street fight. The following are natural body weapon targets: eyes, temple, nose, chin, back of neck, front of neck, solar plexus, ribs, groin, thighs, knees, and shins.

Target recognition requires that you maintain a *complete* visual picture of your adversary (i.e., head, torso, and limbs). One of the biggest mistakes that you can make during a street fight is to gaze or stare into your opponent's eyes. Looking steadily into the assailant's eyes will significantly restrict your ability to recognize targets during a fight.

Target Selection

A highly skilled fighter will never strike his opponent with reckless abandon. His swift blows are strategically calculated, and he is a true maven of target selection. Target selection is the cognitive process of selecting the appropriate anatomical target to attack in a street fight. It is predicated on three important factors:

1. *Proximity of opponent*—how far the opponent is from your natural body weapon, technique, or weapon.
2. *Positioning of opponent*—exactly where the opponent is positioned and at what angle and height.
3. *Use of force*—the amount of force (non-deadly or deadly) that is legally warranted for this particular self-defense situation.

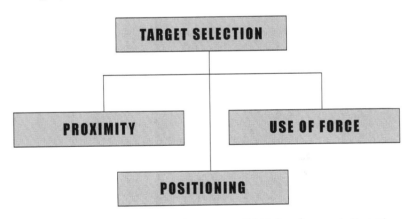

Selecting the appropriate target to strike in a street fight is based on proximity, positioning, and the use of force justification.

Target Impaction

Target impaction is the physical process of successfully striking the selected anatomical target. Target impaction requires that every blow be delivered with maximum speed and power and minimal telegraphing. Proper attribute development will ensure successful target impact during the course of a street fight.

Target Exploitation

Once you have achieved target impaction, you can implement target exploitation. Target exploitation is a combat attribute that allows you to strategically maximize (through exploitation) your assailant's reaction dynamics during the fight. By the way, target exploitation skills can be applied in both armed and unarmed encounters.

GHOSTING

One of the best ways to avoid staring is by "ghosting" your adversary. Ghosting is the process of mentally eliminating all the facial features on your opponent (particularly his eyes) so that he appears completely faceless. Besides eliminating gazing, ghosting also enhances your ability to pseudospeciate your adversary. Pseudospeciation is the ability to assign inferior and subhuman qualities to a threatening opponent. This psychological strategy is important when launching your first strike, because it will make it psychologically easier for you to attack your adversary with vicious intent and determination. Pseudospeciation is also important because it allows you to unleash your killer instinct while liberating you from the inherent dangers and risks of moral and philosophical apprehension.

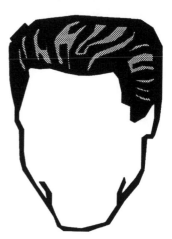

Preceding a first strike and during the delivery of your compound attack, it's important to "ghost" your adversary.

COMBAT ATTRIBUTES

Your preemptive strike must be accompanied by specific combat attributes, or unique qualities that enhance your particular tool, technique, or weapon. Combat attributes are divided into one of two categories: cognitive and physical.

Cognitive attributes are the mental properties that enhance your street fighting skills and abilities. Some examples are courageousness, perceptiveness, viciousness, decisiveness, awareness, and the killer instinct. Physical attributes are the physical qualities that enhance your street fighting skills and abilities. Examples of common physical attributes are speed, power, timing, agility, ambidexterity, weapon and technique mastery, and physical fitness.

Although there are well over 100 combat attributes available to a fighter, there are five physical attributes (motor skills) that are necessary to successfully land a preemptive strike: speed, impact power, offensive timing, balance, and non telegraphic movement.

Speed

You have to be fast—*real fast!* That means that your offensive and defensive techniques must move like a flash of lightning. In unarmed street combat, there are two types of speed that should be of concern to you:

1. Mental—the rate at which you can think and employ your cognitive skills (i.e., assessment, awareness, tactical option response) in a self-defense situation.
2. Psychomotor—the rate at which you can move your body (e.g., punching, blocking, evading) in a street fighting situation. It behooves the serious fighter to make every possible attempt to develop his combat speed to the best of his ability.

One of the most effective methods of enhancing the physical speed of your offensive and defensive techniques is to avoid tensing your body and to simply relax your muscles prior to executing your movement. Another way of developing blistering speed is to practice a particular technique *thousands* of times until the psycho motor movement is sharpened and crystallized. Also, proper breathing will optimize psycho motor speed.

Impact Power

In street combat, you want to hit your opponent with the power equivalent of a 12-gauge shotgun. Impact power refers to the amount of force you can generate when striking your opponent's targets.

Contrary to popular belief, punching and kicking power is not simply predicated on size and strength. There are other significant factors, such as power generator mastery, follow-through, and tool velocity that also play a critical role. This explains why a relatively small person can generate devastating power exceeding that of a 200-pound man.

When punching your opponent, remember to put your entire body behind the strike by torquing your hip, shoulder, and foot; aim three inches through your selected target; and allow your blow to temporarily sink into your target.

Offensive Reaction Time

The ability to launch a first strike at the right moment cannot be overstated. You must possess an accurate sense of timing. Timing refers to your ability to execute a technique or movement at the precise moment. There are two types of timing that are used in street combat: defensive reaction time and offensive reaction time.

Defensive reaction time is defined as the elapsed time between the opponent's physical attack and your defensive response to that attack. (For more information on defensive reaction time, please refer to Chapter 3.)

Offensive reaction time refers to the elapsed time between offensive recognition and offensive execution. Your offensive reaction time is the result of three stages (offensive recognition, offensive selection, and offensive execution).

1. *Offensive recognition* is the first stage where you recognize and identify the ability to attack the opponent.
2. *Offensive selection* is the second stage where you immediately select the appropriate offensive tool or technique.
3. *Offensive execution* is the third stage where your body executes the appropriate offensive tool or technique.

Some of the best ways of developing offensive timing are through intense sparring sessions, double-end bag training, and various focus mitt drills. Mental visualization is also another effective method of enhancing your combat timing. Visualizing various first-strike scenarios that require precise timing is ideal for enhancing your skills.

Balance

An effective first strike requires substantial follow-through while maintaining your balance. Balance is your ability to maintain equilibrium while attacking and defending. You can maintain your balance in combat by controlling your center of gravity, mastering body mechanics, and maintaining proper skeletal alignment.

To develop a better sense of balance, exercise your body weapons slowly in front of a mirror so you become acquainted with the different weight distributions, body positions, and mechanics of each particular technique. Also, remember that balance is often lost because of weak body mechanics, poor kinesthetic perception, unnecessary weight shifting, excessive follow-through, and improper skeletal alignment.

Non Telegraphic Movement (Invisible Deployment)

It is critical to not telegraph or forewarn your opponent of your intentions to launch a first strike. Telegraphing means inadvertently making your offensive intentions known to your adversary. In street combat, you must possess "clean" body mechanics that don't inform your adversary of your combat agenda. Basically, all of your movements have to be non telegraphic.

There are many forms of telegraphing that need to be purged from your arsenal: staring at your selected target, chambering your arm back before striking, clenching your fists prior to punching, tensing any part of your torso, grinning or opening your mouth, widening your eyes or raising your eyebrows, and taking a sudden, deep breath.

COMPOUND ATTACK AND OFFENSIVE FLOW

It will take more than just a preemptive strike to enervate your adversary. To complete the job, you will almost always have to initiate a strategic compound attack. A compound attack is what immediately follows your first strike, and it's defined as the logical sequence of two or more tools strategically thrown in succession. The objective is to take the fight out of the assailant and the assailant out of the fight by destroying his defenses with a flurry of full-speed, full-force strikes.

Based on speed, power, target selection, and target exploitation, the compound attack also requires calculation, precision, and clarity. To maximize your compound attack, you must have a thorough knowledge and awareness of the anatomical targets presented by your adversary. Unless your assailant is in full body armor, there are always targets. It is simply a question of your selecting them and striking quickly with the appropriate body weapons.

When you proceed with the compound attack, always maintain the offensive flow. The offensive flow is a progression of continuous offensive movements designed to neutralize or, in some cases, terminate your adversary. The key is to have each strike flow smoothly and efficiently from one to the next without causing you to lose ground. Subjecting your adversary to an offensive flow is especially effective because it taxes his nervous system, thereby dramatically lengthening his defensive reaction time.

In a real-life street fight it's critical that you always keep the offensive pressure on until your opponent is completely neutralized. Always remember that letting your offensive flow stagnate, *even for a second*, will open you up to numerous dangers and risks.

Proper breathing is another substantial element of the compound attack, and there is one simple rule that should be followed: exhale during the execution phase of your strike and inhale during its retraction phase. Above all, *never* hold your breath when delivering several consecutive blows. Doing so could lead to dizziness and fainting, among other complications.

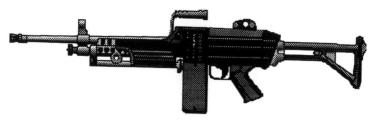

In many ways, your offensive skills must be comparable with a high-powered machine gun. During the course of your compound attack, it's imperative that you overwhelm your adversary by showering him with a barrage of rapid, successive blows designed to both injure him and demolish his defenses. Have you developed the necessary firepower to neutralize your enemy?

YOU DON'T HAVE MUCH TIME

Your body can only sustain delivering a compound attack for so long. Initially, your brain will quickly release adrenaline or epinephrine into your blood stream, which will fuel your fighting and enhance your strength and power. This lethal boost of energy is known as an *adrenaline dump*. However, your ability to exert and maintain this maximum effort in a compound attack will last no more than 30 to 60 seconds if you are in above-average shape. If the fight continues after that, your strength and speed may drop by as much as 50 percent below normal. When all is said and done, you don't have much time in a street fight, so the battle needs to be won fast before your energy runs out!

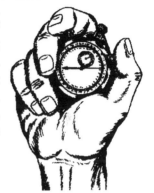

DON'T FORGET TO RELOCATE!

Subsequent to your compound attack, immediately move to a new location by flanking your adversary. This tactic is known as *relocating*. Based on the principles of strategy, movement, and surprise, relocating dramatically enhances your safety by making it difficult for your adversary to identify your position after you have attacked him. Remember, if your opponent doesn't know exactly where you are, he won't be able to effectively counterattack.

ACTUATE RECOVERY BREATHING

Implementing an explosive compound attack will often leave you winded. Because of the volatile nature of street combat, even highly conditioned fighters will show signs of oxygen debt. Hence it's important to employ recovery breathing, the active process of quickly restoring your breathing to its normal state. It requires taking long, deep breaths in a controlled rhythm while avoiding rapid, short gasping. Wind sprints are great for improving your recovery breathing. Consider adding them to your regular training program.

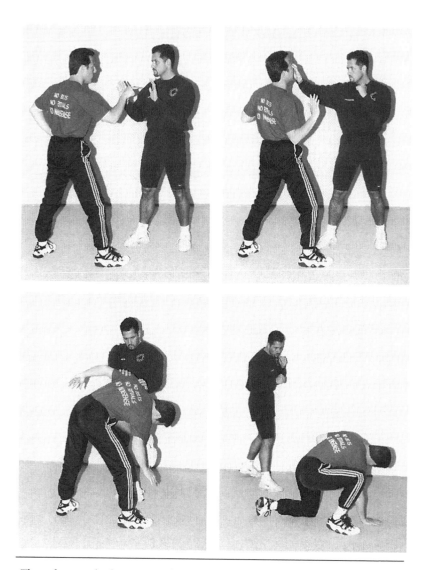

These photographs demonstrate the relocation tactic.

GEMINI PRINCIPLE

Before a first strike is delivered there is almost always going to be some form of dialogue between you and the opponent. This is when the "Gemini" principle should be used. The Gemini principle is the strategic and deceptive use of both verbal and nonverbal skills that enables you to successfully launch a preemptive strike. As in the Gemini zodiac, you need to summon the "dark twin" of your personality to effectively perform this type of disingenuous behavior.

Once you assume your first-strike stance, your next objective is to psychologically manipulate or "soften" your adversary by speaking to him in a calm and unresisting tone of voice, telling him that you have no intentions of fighting. The key is to prolong the opponent's thought process and momentarily distract him. Once he takes the bait and "lowers his guard," launch your first strike and keep the pressure on until he is thoroughly incapacitated (generally the best time to strike your opponent is while you're talking to him, preferably in the form of a question).

This form of disingenuous vocalization requires a calm demeanor, precise timing, and a good bit of acting on your part. When conducting the Gemini principle be certain not to get locked into a dialogue with your adversary. Remember, dialogue is simply a tool that is used to slacken an opponent's defenses and provide you with a window of opportunity. **WARNING:** *Like any tactic or strategy, the Gemini principle can backfire if not properly and confidently employed.*

FIFTH-COLUMN TACTIC

You can also deploy the first-strike strategy when a significant other (e.g., close friend, spouse, acquaintance, co-worker, partner) is physically threatened by an adversary. I call this the *fifth-column tactic.*

As with the Gemini principle, the fifth-column tactic is the strategic and deceptive application of both verbal and nonverbal skills that permit you to successfully launch a preemptive strike. What follows are six principles of the fifth-column tactic:

1. When the hostile and threatening adversary initially confronts your friend, you should psychologically manipulate and soften the opponent by taking his side in the argument, regardless of how ridiculous his position might be.
2. Always appear nonthreatening and yielding to the adversary by assuming your unaggressive first-strike stance.
3. Speak to the adversary in a calm, unresisting tone and be certain to tell him that you and your friend have no intentions of fighting.
4. Distract and confuse the adversary by becoming angry with your friend. Raise your voice and castigate your friend for quarreling with the adversary (this will require a good bit of acting on your part).
5. While verbally sympathizing with the opponent, you should subtly reposition yourself to the most advantageous striking position.
6. Once you have attained the ideal striking position and your partner is out of the line of fire, launch your first strike at the adversary and keep the pressure on until he is thoroughly incapacitated.
Remember, never deliver a first strike unless it's legally warranted and justified in the eyes of the law.

FEAR MANAGEMENT

Although you have the strategic advantage of launching a first strike against your opponent, the element of fear or anxiety may still be present. Fear is a strong and unpleasant emotional reaction to a real or perceived threat. If uncontrolled, fear leads to panic, and panic is disastrous in a street fight. To prevent fear and anxiety from dominating you, it is critical that you understand its dynamics: the fight-or-flight response.

What Is Fight-or-Flight Response?

Whenever a person feels threatened, certain physiological changes occur. They begin in the brain when the hypothalamus sends strong impulses to the pituitary gland, causing it to release a hormone (ACTH) that stimulates the adrenal glands to release other hormones into the bloodstream.

Ultimately every nerve and muscle are involved. This adrenaline will cause an increased heart rate with a corresponding increase in respiration and blood pressure. Your muscles will tense up, you will start to sweat, and your mouth will become dry. Furthermore, your digestive system will shut down to allow a better supply of blood to the muscles. Your hair will stand on end (piloerection). Your pupils will enlarge to improve vision, and your hands and limbs will begin to tremble. You are now in the fight-or-flight mode.

For untrained fighters, the fight-or-flight response is debilitating. They often panic and freeze at the critical moment. Therefore, it is vitally important that you learn to control and command the fight-or-flight response to make it work for you and not against you.

First, you must accept the fact that the fight-or-flight response is natural and unavoidable. In fact, it's Mother Nature's best way of helping you survive a street fight. You've got to take advantage of this assistance by using the energy of the adrenaline surge to augment your compound attack and awaken your killer instinct. Actually, the killer instinct burns on the fuel of adrenaline, and it can be a very powerful source of energy. Properly channeled, this destructiveness will exceed that of your enemy and overwhelm him.

Second, you can harness the fight-or-flight response by preparing yourself mentally and physically for street combat. Developing and refining the psychological and physiological tools of combat will improve your confidence. In turn, this self-confidence leads to an inner calm. Inner calm is the mental environment that permits you to perform at your peak.

Your mental and physical preparation involves learning and mastering the skills, techniques, and tactics of street combat. The only way to achieve these skills is through qualified instruction and consistent practice. This approach will instill psychological preparedness. Once you begin to understand what a street fight entails, you can expand your training to regularly visualizing various fights and altercations and the necessary control over the fight-or-flight syndrome.

KILLER INSTINCT

Techniques alone will not equip you for the rigors of a life-threatening street fight. It is imperative that you possess a combative mentality to channel a destructiveness that exceeds your opponent's. The bottom line is that you must be a cold, vicious animal when fighting your adversary. This mind-set results from mastery of the killer instinct. The killer instinct is a ferocious, combative mentality that surges to one's consciousness and turns him into a focused fighter free of fear, anger, and apprehension.

There are 15 characteristics that harmoniously integrate to create the killer instinct:

1. Clear, lucid thinking
2. Heightened situational awareness
3. Adrenaline surge
4. Physical mobilization
5. Psychomotor control
6. Absence of distractions
7. Tunnel vision
8. Courage
9. Tactical implementation
10. Lack of emotion
11. Breath control

12. Ability to pseudospeciate
13. Viciousness
14. Pain tolerance
15. Habituation to violence

Visualization techniques and crisis rehearsal methods are just a few techniques used to forge and discipline this extraordinary source of strength and energy.

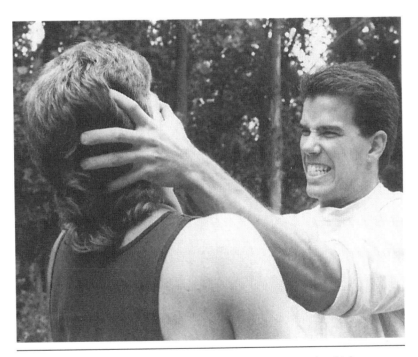

There is a deadly power coiled deep within each of us. It is a natural and inherent instinct to struggle and fight against the grim reaper's call. This power is the killer instinct—a cold primal power that can surge to the surface and turn a calm and mundane person into a vicious animal that is free of fear, anger, and apprehension.

FIRST STRIKE

CHAPTER 3

WHEN THINGS GO BAD, IT'S TIME FOR DEFENSE

DEFENSE IS A TEMPORARY SETBACK

One unfortunate fact of life is that sometimes things do not always go as planned. In unarmed combat, there is always the possibility that your first strike will be thwarted and your opponent will counter swiftly with an attack of his own. In such a case you will have no choice but to temporarily resort to defensive tactics.

Defense should be looked at as a temporary setback that will eventually allow you to counter with offensive viciousness. A good defensive structure requires mastery of the following four tools: blocks, parries, slipping, and footwork. I know firsthand that all of these defensive techniques work effectively against boxers, street fighters, and martial artists of all styles and backgrounds. However, before I can discuss the specific defensive tools, it's important to address defensive reaction time and its implication in a street fight.

HOW TO MINIMIZE DEFENSIVE REACTION TIME

Defensive reaction time is defined as the elapsed time between the assailant's physical attack (e.g., punch, kick, throat grab) and your defensive response to that attack (e.g., block, parry, evasion movement). Your defensive reaction time is the result of three stages (defensive recognition, defensive selection, and defensive execution).

1. **Defensive recognition** is the first stage where you recognize and identify that an attack has occurred.
2. **Defensive selection** is the second stage where you immediately select the appropriate defensive tool, technique, or response.
3. **Defensive execution** is the third and final stage where your body executes the appropriate defensive tool, technique, or response.

When it comes to street combat, your objective is to try to reduce or minimize your defensive reaction time as much as possible. There are several ways to accomplish this. First, be able to read advance information about the opponent's attack. This is referred to as *telegraphic cognizance*. For example, this occurs when your adversary chambers his arm back prior to delivering a haymaker punch.

Second, limit your number of defensive responses to a particular type of attack. For example, if your opponent attacks with a haymaker punch to your head, you should have only *one specific* defensive response programmed. In this instance, you would use a mid-block to intercept the threatening blow.

Third, all of your defensive responses should be natural and executed in a simple fashion. Again, in the case of the haymaker, not

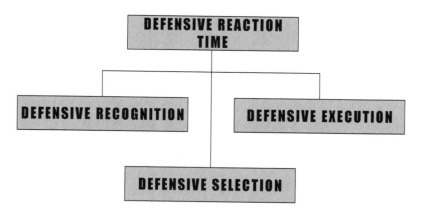

Defensive reaction time is the result of three stages: defensive recognition, defensive selection, and defensive execution.

only would you execute a mid-block, but you would also situate it on the same side of the opponent's attack (this is referred to as mirror-image blocking).

Fourth, practice, practice, practice! Your defensive responses must be practiced over and over again until they become second nature. Therefore, you'll need to set aside some time from your busy schedule, and this will require a bit of discipline and planning on your part.

BLOCKS

Blocks are defensive techniques designed to intercept your assailant's circular attacks. Blocks are executed by placing a non vital body part between the assailant's strike and your anatomical body target. There are three primary blocks with which you need to be proficient. They include high blocks, mid-blocks, and elbow blocks. To maximize the execution of your hand blocks, remember to always keep your hands open.

DON'T FORGET!

You can significantly reduce defensive reaction time by applying some of the following strategies:

- Recognize advance information about your opponent's attack.
- Limit your number of defensive options to a particular attack.
- Make your defensive response natural and simple.
- Practice, practice, practice!

High Block

The high block is used to defend against overhead blows. To execute the lead high block, simply raise your lead arm up and extend your forearm out and above your head. Be careful not to position your arm where your head is exposed. Make certain that your hand is open and not clenched. This will increase the surface area of your block and provide a quick counterattack. The mechanics for the lead high block are the same as for the rear high block. Raise your rear arm up and extend your forearm out and above your head.

Mid-Block

The mid-block is specifically used to defend against circular blows to your head or upper torso. To perform the block, raise either your right or left arm at approximately 90 degrees while simultaneously pronating (rotating) it into the direction of the strike. Make contact with the belly of your forearm at the assailant's wrist or forearm. This movement will provide maximum structural integrity for the blocking tool. Make certain that your hand is held open to increase the surface area of your block. When performing the mid-block, be certain to time the rotation of your arm with the attack. Don't forget that the mid-block has both height (up and down) and width (in and out) fluctuations that are relative to the characteristics of the assailant's blow. Remember, once you deliver the block, immediately counter.

Elbow Block

The elbow block is used to stop circular blows to your midsection, such as uppercuts, shovel hooks, and even hook kicks. To execute the elbow block, drop your elbow and simultaneously twist your body toward your centerline. Be certain to keep your elbow perpendicular to the floor and keep your hands relaxed and close to your chest. The elbow block can be used on both the right and left sides.

PARRIES

The parry is a quick, forceful slap that redirects your assailant's linear strike (jabs, lead straights, and rear crosses). There are two general types of parries, horizontal and vertical, and both can be

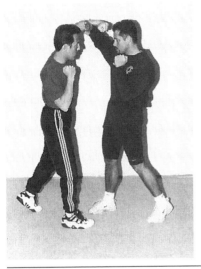

The high block.

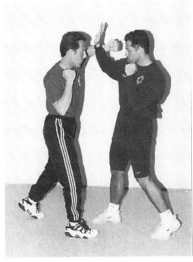

The mid-block.

executed with the right and left hands.

Horizontal Parry

To properly execute a horizontal parry from a fighting stance, move your lead hand horizontally across your body (centerline) to deflect and redirect the assailant's punch. Immediately return to your guard position. Be certain to make contact with the palm of your hand. With sufficient training, you can effectively incorporate the horizontal parry into your slipping maneuvers.

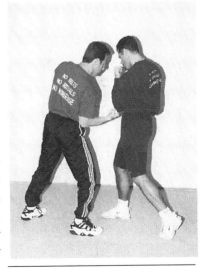

The elbow block.

BE PREPARED FOR THE BEST AND THE WORST

Defensive competency requires you to be adequately prepared to defend against myriad adversaries, including poorly skilled opponents. For example, you must be capable of defending against a clean, tight hook punch as well as a sloppy, awkward haymaker. This reminds me of the saying, "Professionals are predictable, but the world is filled with amateurs." Don't make the tragic mistake of thinking that all opponents will attack you in the same fashion. Remember, there are as many styles of fighting as there are ways of thinking.

Vertical Parry

To execute a vertical parry, from a fighting stance, move your hand vertically down your body (centerline) to deflect and redirect the assailant's blow. Once again, don't forget to counterattack your assailant. **CAUTION:** *Do not parry with your fingers. The fingers provide no structural integrity, and they can be jammed or broken easily.*

SLIPPING

Slipping is a quick defensive maneuver that permits you to

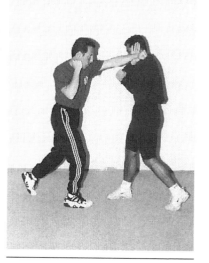

The horizontal parry.

avoid an assailant's linear blow (e.g., jab, lead straight, rear cross) without stepping out of range. Safe and effective slipping requires precise timing and is accomplished by quickly snapping the head and upper torso sideways (right or left) or backward to avoid the oncoming blow. One of the greatest advantages to slipping is that it frees your hands so that you can simultaneously counter your attacker. There are three ways to slip: right, left, and back.

Slipping Right

Begin from a fighting stance and quickly sway your head and upper torso to the right to avoid the assailant's blow. Quickly counter or return to the starting position.

Slipping Left

Start from a fighting stance and quickly sway your head and upper torso to the left to avoid the assailant's linear blow. Quickly counter or return to the starting position.

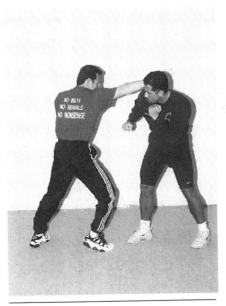

Slipping requires precise timing.

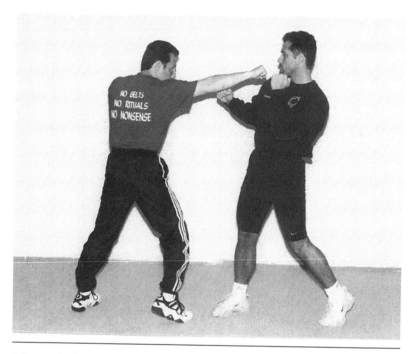

The snap back.

Slipping Back (or the Snap Back)

Begin from a fighting stance and quickly snap your head back enough to avoid being hit. Quickly counter or return to the starting position.

FOOTWORK

The final, and probably most important, component of defense is footwork. In defense, footwork allows you to disengage quickly from the range of attack. (For more detailed information about footwork, reread the section on mobility and footwork in Chapter 2.)

A QUICK WORD ABOUT GROUND FIGHTING

Regardless of how skilled you might be with your defensive techniques, there is still a very strong possibility that your adversary will take the street fight to the ground. Actually, it is estimated that nine out of ten fights go to the ground. Therefore, it's of paramount importance that you equip yourself with the knowledge, skills, and attitude necessary to prevail in a ground fight.

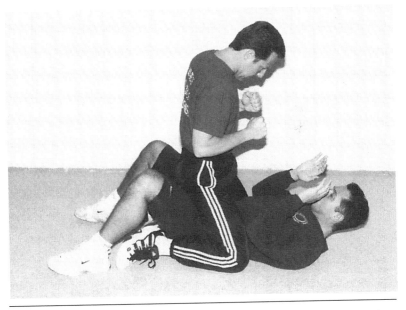

Approximately 90 percent of all street fights end up on the ground. Do you know how to ground fight?

HOW WILL YOU REACT WHEN HIT?

Now is the time to give serious thought to how you will react if you are hit by the assailant. I know of several fighters who just fall to the floor and give up even though they are not completely incapacitated. If you are hit in a street fight, it's critical that you keep fighting. Never give up! Remember, if you are able to comprehend that you've been hit, then you're capable of fighting, provided that you are psychologically conditioned not to throw in the towel.

AVOID THE OSTRICH DEFENSE

Throughout my years of teaching thousands of students, I've noticed that one of the most common mistakes a frightened fighter can make when he's bombarded by blows is to close his eyes or reflexively drop his head. This is the "ostrich defense," and it can get you killed in a matter of seconds. With the ostrich defense, the practitioner will quickly look away from that which he fears (e.g., a punch, kick, strike) in hopes that it will go away. His fallacious thinking is, *If I can't see it, it can't hurt me.*

One of the best ways of eliminating the ostrich-defense response is to experience full-contact sparring wearing protective headgear. During full-contact sessions, you must make a conscious effort to keep your head erect and your eyes open amid flying blows. If you do get hit, don't panic. Just keep moving, maintain proper breathing, apply the appropriate defensive response, and counterattack when the opportunity presents itself. Acquiring this necessary skill will require a considerable amount of training, but it can be accomplished.

CHAPTER 4

FIRST-STRIKE TOOLS

"While we stop to think, we often miss our opportunity."

—Publilius Syrus
1st century B.C.

Now that you're acquainted with the first-strike prerequisites, it's time to learn the actual tools. First-strike tools are specific offensive techniques designed to initiate a preemptive strike against your adversary. Unlike the other offensive tools and techniques in your cache, the following preemptive strikes were chosen because they are quick, destructive, and virtually non-telegraphic. Let's start with the vertical kick.

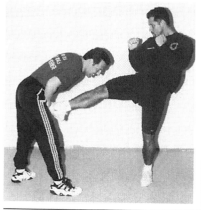 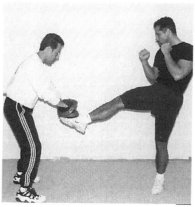

The vertical kick.

The focus mitts are ideal for developing a powerful and lightning-quick vertical kick.

VERTICAL KICK

The vertical kick is delivered off your lead leg and travels on a vertical path to the assailant's groin. To execute the vertical kick, maintain your balance while quickly shifting your weight to your rear leg and simultaneously raising your lead leg vertically into the assailant's groin. Once you make contact, quickly force your leg back to the ground. Keep your supporting leg bent for balance. Contact should always be made with the instep of your lead foot. Avoid the tendency to snap your knee as you deliver the kick.

Vertical-Kick Training Exercise

The best piece of training equipment for developing the vertical kick is a pair of focus mitts. Begin by having your training partner hold the two mitts at kicking range. From a right stance (your right food forward), keep your body relaxed and deliver 25 rapid and powerful vertical kicks into the focus mitt. Maintain your balance and proper form throughout the entire movement. Switch to a left stance and execute 25 more repetitions.

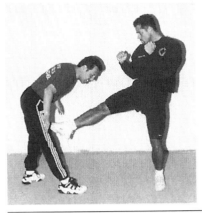

The push kick.

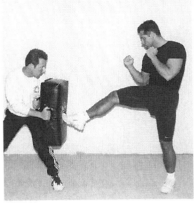

Make certain to brace the striking shield against your body when holding it for your training partner.

PUSH KICK

The push kick is another efficient first-strike tool that is delivered from your lead leg. To execute the kick, quickly shift your weight to your rear leg and simultaneously raise your lead leg. Thrust the ball of your foot into the assailant's groin, quadriceps, knee, or shin. Quickly drop your leg to the ground. Make certain to keep your supporting leg bent for balance.

Push-Kick Training Exercise

The striking shield is your best bet for sharpening the push kick. Begin by having your training partner hold the foam shield at kicking range, approximately waist level.

From a right-lead stance, keep your body relaxed and deliver 25 quick, powerful push kicks into the shield. Take your time and pause between each repetition. Switch to a left stance and execute 25 more reps.

FINGER JAB

The finger jab is a quick, non-telegraphic strike executed from your lead arm. Contact is made with your fingertips. To execute the finger jab properly, quickly shoot your arm out and back. Don't tense your muscles before the execution of the strike. Just relax and send it out. Targets for the finger jab are the assailant's eyes. Don't forget that a finger-jab strike can cause temporary or permanent blindness, severe pain, and shock. Remember, with the finger jab, you want speed, accuracy, and, above all, non-telegraphic movement.

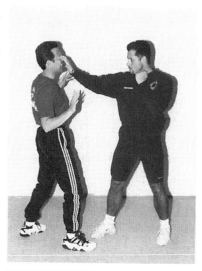

The finger jab.

Finger-Jab Training Exercise

An X-ray chart is ideal for developing a lightning-quick finger jab. To begin, have your training partner hold the chart at the punching range, approximately six feet high. From a right stance, deliver 50 quick, non-telegraphic strikes. Take your time with each repetition. Switch to a left stance and execute 50 more reps.

Finger-Jab Training (Exercise 2)

A mannequin head can be used to develop accurate finger-jab strikes. To begin, have your training partner hold the head at the punching range, approximately six feet high. From a right stance, launch 50 quick, non-telegraphic strikes. Once again, take your time with each repetition. Switch to a left stance and execute 50 more reps.

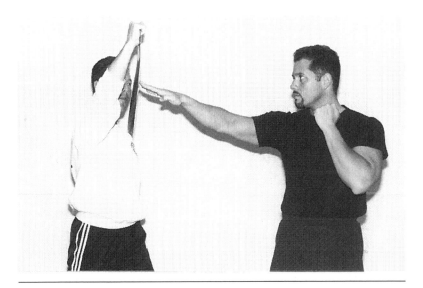

When holding the X-ray chart for your partner, be sure to keep it to the side of your body and away from your face.

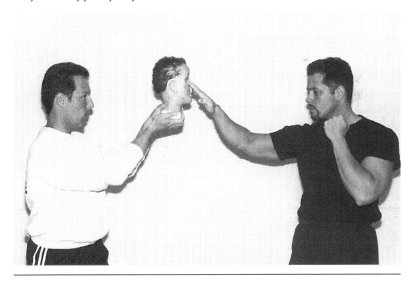

A mannequin head is unsurpassed as a training tool for developing accurate finger-jab strikes.

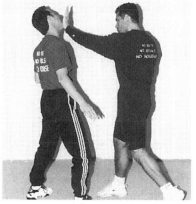 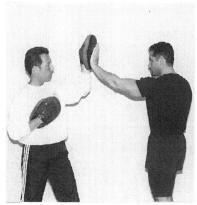

The rear palm-heel strike.

The correct method of holding the focus mitts for a palm-heel strike is to make certain they are held perpendicular to the floor.

REAR PALM-HEEL STRIKE

The rear palm-heel strike is a powerful open-hand linear blow. Contact is made with the heel of your palm with the fingers pointing up. Targets include your assailant's nose and chin. When delivering the blow, be certain to torque your shoulder, hips, and foot in the direction of the strike. Make certain that your arm extends straight out and that the heel of your palm makes contact with either the assailant's nose or chin. Remember to retract your arm along the same line in which you initiated the strike.

Rear Palm-Heel Training Exercise

The focus mitt should be used to develop powerful palm-heel strikes. Begin by having your training partner hold the mitt at the punching range. From a right stance, launch 25 powerful, non-telegraphic strikes. Once again, take your time with each repetition. Switch to a left stance and execute 25 more reps.

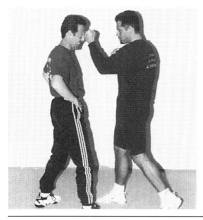 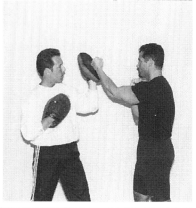

The rear vertical hammer fist (short arc).

When developing the rear vertical hammer fist (short arc), be certain to hold the focus mitt at a 45-degree angle from the floor.

REAR VERTICAL HAMMER FIST

The rear vertical hammer fist (short arc) is a quick and powerful strike that is delivered at close range to the adversary. Your target is the assailant's nose. To deliver the vertical hammer fist, begin by raising your fist with your elbow flexed. Quickly whip your clenched fist down in a vertical line onto the bridge of your assailant's nose. Remember to keep your elbow bent on impact and maintain your balance throughout execution.

Rear Vertical Hammer-Fist Training Exercise

The rear vertical hammer fist (short arc) is developed on the focus mitt. Start by having your training partner hold the mitt at the punching range, with the mitt angled at approximately 45 degrees.

From a right stance, execute 25 quick, non-telegraphic strikes. Be certain to take your time with each repetition. Switch to a left stance and execute 25 more reps.

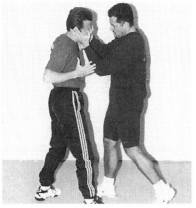 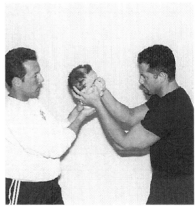

The double-thumb gouge.   *Always attack the mannequin head with vicious determination.*

DOUBLE-THUMB GOUGE

The double-thumb gouge is a grappling-range tactic that can produce devastating results. This tactic can be delivered when either standing or fighting on the ground.

To perform the gouge, place both hands on the assailant's face. Stabilize your hands by wrapping your bottom fingers around both sides of your assailant's jaw. Immediately drive both your thumbs into the assailant's eye sockets. Maintain and increase forceful pressure. The double-thumb gouge can cause temporary or permanent blindness, shock, and unconsciousness. **WARNING:** *The double-thumb gouge should only be used in life-and-death situations! Be certain that it is legally warranted and justified.*

Double-Thumb Gouge Training Exercise

Although the double-thumb gouge is a low-maintenance tool that requires very little practice to master, it nevertheless should be sharpened from time to time. The best piece of training equipment to sharpen this technique on is a mannequin head.

Start by having your partner hold the head at the punching range, about six feet high. From a right stance, execute 15 powerful gouges. Remember to take your time with each repetition. Switch to a left stance and execute 15 more reps.

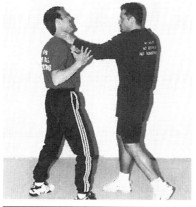 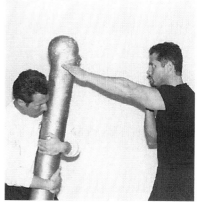

The rear web hand strike.

Take your time when training on the choking dummy and progressively build the force of your rear web-hand strikes.

REAR WEB-HAND STRIKE

The rear web-hand strike is a grappling-range technique that can produce devastating results. Depending on the amount of force, a strike to the throat can cause gagging, excruciating pain, loss of breath, nausea, and possibly death.

To perform the strike, simultaneously separate your thumb from your index finger and quickly drive the web of your hand into the adversary's throat. Be certain to keep your hand stiff with your palm down. Once contact is made, quickly retract your hand to the starting position. **WARNING:** *The web-hand strike should only be used in life-and-death situations! Be certain that it is legally warranted and justified.*

Rear Web-Hand Training Exercise

The choking dummy should be used to develop the rear web-hand strike. Begin by having your training partner hold the dummy at the punching range, approximately six feet high. From a right stance, execute 20 non-telegraphic strikes. Remember to follow through your target. Switch to a left stance and execute 20 more reps.

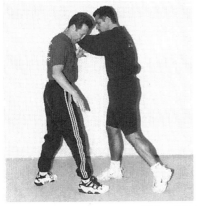

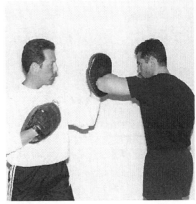

The rear horizontal elbow.

When helping your partner develop the rear horizontal elbow, hold the focus mitts with sufficient resistance.

REAR HORIZONTAL ELBOW

The rear horizontal elbow is a devastating weapon used in grappling range. It is explosive, deceptive, and very difficult to stop. The rear horizontal-elbow strike travels horizontally to the assailant's face.

To perform the strike, quickly rotate your hips and shoulders horizontally into your target. Your palms should be facing downward with your hand next to the side of your head. The striking surface is the elbow point.

Rear Horizontal-Elbow Training Exercise

The focus mitt should be used to develop and refine the rear horizontal elbow. Begin by having your training partner hold the mitt at grappling range. From a right stance, launch 25 powerful, non-telegraphic strikes. Once again, take your time with each repetition. Switch to a left stance and execute 25 more reps. Don't forget to follow through your target.

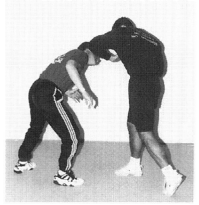 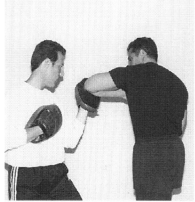

The rear diagonal elbow (traveling downward).

The rear diagonal elbow will take significant time to master. Be patient and it will come.

REAR DIAGONAL ELBOW

The rear diagonal-elbow strike travels diagonally downward to the assailant's face, throat, or body. It can be delivered from either the right or left side of the body. To execute the strike, rotate your elbow back, up, and over while quickly whipping it down to your desired target. Bend your knees as your body descends with the strike. Your palm should be facing away from you when making contact. The striking surface is the elbow point.

Rear Diagonal-Elbow Training Exercise

The rear diagonal elbow is a powerful downward strike that is best developed on the focus mitt. Begin by having your training partner hold the mitt at grappling range, approximately five and a half feet high. Make certain that your partner angles the mitt at 45 degrees.

From a right stance, launch 25 powerful, non-telegraphic strikes. Once again, take your time with each repetition. Switch to a left stance and execute 25 more reps.

ADVANCED FIRST-STRIKE TOOLS

Now that you've completed the first-strike arsenal, it's time to address the advanced first-strike tools. Advanced first-strike tools are offensive techniques specifically used to initiate a first strike against multiple opponents. The following three tools should be included in your toolbox of weapons: side kick (to the flank), horizontal hammer fist, and horizontal knife hand.

Side Kick (to the Flank)

The side kick is a powerful linear kick executed from either the rear or lead leg. Contact is made with the heel. To execute either the lead-side kick, shift your weight back, pivot your rear foot, and simultaneously raise and thrust your lead hip and leg into the assailant. Remember that you must pivot your rear foot to facilitate proper skeletal alignment (shoulder, hip, and heel alignment). The side kick is targeted for either the assailant's hip, thigh, knee, or shinbone.

Side-Kick Training Exercise

The shin guard is used to develop the side kick. Since the side kick is best delivered to the flank, begin with your training partner standing to your right side at kicking range.

From a right stance, launch 20 powerful, non-telegraphic kicks. Once again, take your time with each repetition. Switch to a left stance and execute 20 more reps.

Horizontal Hammer Fist

The horizontal hammer fist is a powerful strike that is delivered horizontally to the assailant's nose. To deliver the horizontal hammer fist, simultaneously torque your shoulder, hip, and leg horizontally into the direction of the blow. Remember to keep your elbow bent on impact and maintain your balance throughout execution. **CAUTION:** *Never deliver a hammer-fist strike with a straight arm. This will rob you of speed and power and possibly cause a severe elbow strain.*

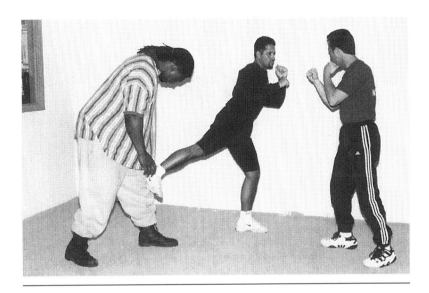

The side kick.

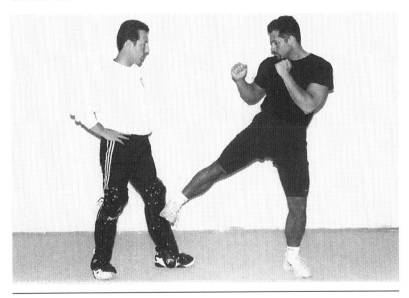

Shin guards can be purchased at any sporting goods store for a reasonable price. However, make certain to buy the ones that cover your entire leg.

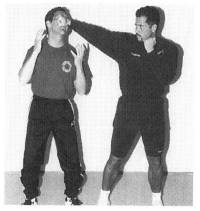 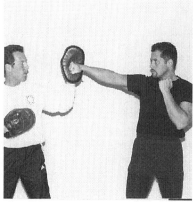

The horizontal hammer fist.

When holding the mitts for the horizontal hammer fist, be sure to keep your elbow slightly bent.

Horizontal Hammer-Fist Training Exercise

The horizontal hammer fist is developed on the focus mitt. Since this strike is delivered to the flank, have your training partner stand to your right side at punching range.

From a right stance, launch 20 powerful, non-telegraphic blows. Once again, take your time with each repetition. Be certain to always turn and look at your target as you whip the blow to your side. Switch to a left stance and execute 20 more reps.

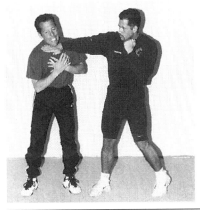 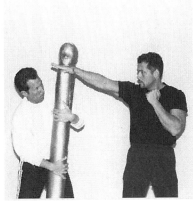

The horizontal knife hand.

When developing the horizontal knife hand, accuracy is everything.

Horizontal Knife Hand

The horizontal knife-hand strike is another tool that can be delivered in both grappling and punching ranges. It can be delivered from both the lead and rear sides. To deliver the horizontal knife hand properly, quickly whip the edge of your hand across and into the adversary's target. Be certain to follow through the target.

Horizontal Knife-Hand Training Exercise

The horizontal knife hand is developed on the choking dummy. Since this strike is delivered to the flank, have your training partner stand to your right side at punching range.

From a right stance, launch 20 powerful, non-telegraphic blows into the throat region of the dummy. Once again, take your time with each repetition. Be certain to always turn and look at your target as you whip the blow to your side. Switch to a left stance and execute 20 more reps.

CHAPTER 5

SECONDARY-STRIKE TOOLS

*"He that has gone so far as to cut the claws of the lion will not feel himself quite
secure until he has also drawn his teeth."*

—Charles Caleb Colton
1825

Secondary-strike tools are offensive techniques that are executed immediately after your first strike. The following 12 techniques compose your compound attack arsenal. We'll begin with the hook kick.

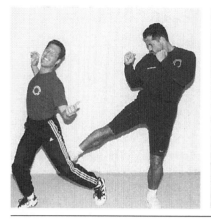 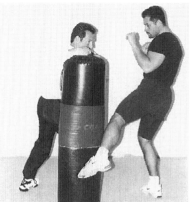

The hook kick.

HOOK KICK

The hook kick is a circular kick that is thrown from your rear leg. Contact is made with either your instep or shinbone. To execute the hook kick, step at a 45-degree angle and simultaneously twist and drive your rear leg and hip into your assailant's target. Make certain to pivot your base foot and follow through your target. When executing the hook kick, either aim for your assailant's knee or drive your shin into the assailant's common peroneal nerve (approximately four inches above the knee area). This will collapse and temporarily immobilize the assailant's leg. Keep in mind that if you strike the knee you can cause permanent damage to the cartilage, ligaments, tendons, and bones.

Hook-Kick Training Exercise

You can develop a powerful hook kick on the kicking cylinder. From a right fighting stance, execute 25 explosive hook kicks. Take your time with each repetition. Be certain that your shinbone penetrates through the bag. Next, switch to a left stance and execute 25 more.

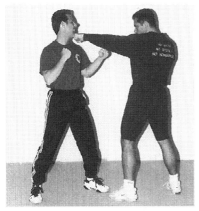 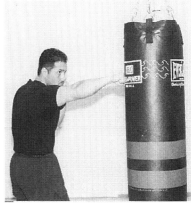

The lead straight.

LEAD STRAIGHT

The lead straight is a linear punch thrown from your lead arm, and contact is made with the center knuckle. To execute the lead straight, quickly twist your lead leg, hip, and shoulder forward. Snap your blow into the assailant's target and return to the starting position. A common mistake is to throw the punch and let it deflect to the side. Targets for the lead straight include the nose, chin, and solar plexus.

Lead-Straight Training Exercise

The heavy bag is by far the best piece of training equipment for developing the lead straight. To begin, start from a right fighting stance and launch 25 punishing blows into the bag. Next, switch to a left stance and deliver 25 more.

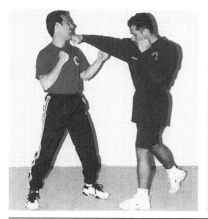 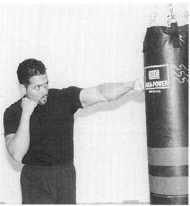

The rear cross.

REAR CROSS

The rear cross is the most powerful linear tool in your unarmed arsenal. This punch travels in a straight direction to your assailant's nose, chin, or solar plexus. Proper waist twisting and weight transfer are of paramount importance to the rear cross. You must shift your weight from your rear foot to your lead leg as you throw the punch. You can generate bone-crushing force by torquing your rear foot, hip, and shoulder into the direction of the blow. To maximize the impact of the punch, make certain that your fist is positioned horizontally. Avoid overextending the blow or exposing your chin during its execution.

Rear-Cross Training Exercise

Once again, the heavy bag is your best tool for sharpening your rear cross. To begin, start from a right stance and drive 25 blows into the bag. Next, switch your stance and execute 25 more.

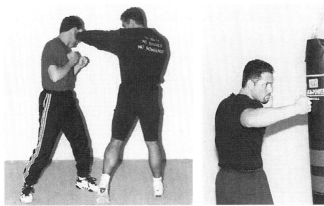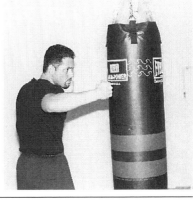

The lead hook punch.

LEAD HOOK PUNCH

The lead hook punch is one of the most difficult to master. To execute the punch properly, you must maintain the correct wrist, forearm, and shoulder alignment. When delivering the strike, be certain that your arm is bent at least 90 degrees and that your wrist and forearm are kept straight throughout the movement.

To execute the lead hook punch, quickly and smoothly raise your elbow so that your arm is parallel to the ground while simultaneously torquing your shoulder, hip, and foot into the direction of the blow. As you throw the punch, be certain that your fist is positioned vertically. Never position your fist horizontally when throwing a hook: this inferior hand placement can cause a sprained or broken wrist. Avoid chambering or cocking the blow and excessive follow-through.

Lead Hook-Punch Training Exercise

Bone-crushing hook punches are best developed on the hook bag. Begin from a right fighting stance and launch 25 explosive blows into the bag. Keep your chin tucked down and be certain to keep your wrist straight during the execution of the punch. Next, switch to a left stance and deliver 25 more.

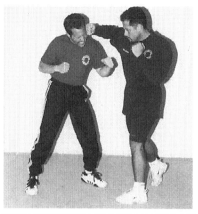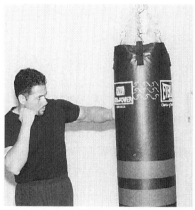

The rear hook punch.

REAR HOOK PUNCH

The rear hook punch is one of the most devastating blows in your arsenal. As with the lead hook, it will take considerable time to master. When delivering the rear hook punch, you must maintain correct wrist, forearm, and shoulder alignment. Once again, your arm must be bent at least 90 degrees while your wrist and forearm are kept straight throughout the movement.

To execute the rear hook punch, quickly and smoothly raise your elbow so that your arm is parallel to the ground while simultaneously torquing your rear shoulder, hip, and foot into the direction of the blow. As you throw the punch, be certain that your fist is positioned vertically.

Rear Hook-Punch Training Exercise

The rear hook punch should also be developed on the focus mitts. Begin from a right fighting stance and launch 25 explosive rear hooks into the mitts. Always remember to keep your chin tucked down during the delivery of the blow. Next, switch to a left stance and deliver 25 more.

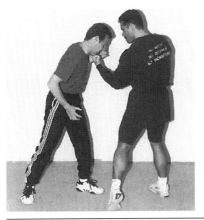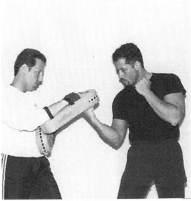

The lead uppercut.

LEAD UPPERCUT

The lead uppercut is a powerful blow that can be delivered in both the punching and grappling ranges. This tool travels in a vertical direction to either the assailant's chin or body, and it is delivered from the lead arm.

To execute the lead uppercut, quickly twist and lift the lead side of your body into the direction of the blow. Make certain that the punch has a short arc and that you avoid any "winding-up" motions.

Lead Uppercut Training Exercise

The lead uppercut should be developed on the focus mitts. Beginning from a right fighting stance, execute 25 punches. Be certain to keep your other hand up and lift with your lead leg. Next, switch to a left fighting stance and deliver 25 more.

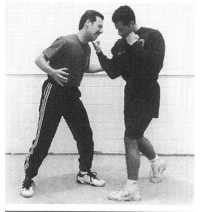 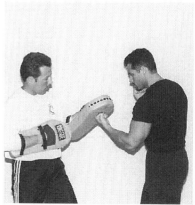

The rear uppercut.

REAR UPPERCUT

The rear uppercut is the mother of all punches. When executed properly it can take any man out of a fight. As does the lead uppercut, it travels in a vertical direction to the adversary's chin or body.

To execute the rear uppercut, quickly twist and lift the rear side of your body into the direction of the blow. Make certain that the blow has a tight arc and that you avoid any telegraphing.

Rear Uppercut Training Exercise

The rear uppercut is also developed on the focus mitts. Beginning from a right fighting stance, execute 25 punches. Next, switch to a left fighting stance and deliver 25 more.

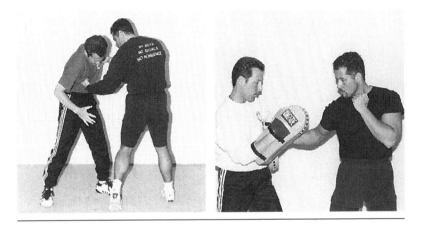

The lead shovel hook.

LEAD SHOVEL HOOK

The lead shovel hook is another powerful punch that travels diagonally into your assailant. To execute the lead shovel hook properly, dip your lead shoulder and simultaneously twist your lead leg and hip into your assailant's target and then drive your entire body into the assailant. Once again, keep balanced and follow through your selected target.

Lead Shovel-Hook Training Exercise

The lead shovel hook can be developed on either the heavy bag or the focus mitts. To begin, start from a right fighting stance and execute 25 powerful blows into the bag. When you are done, switch to a left fighting stance and deliver 25 more.

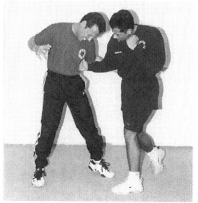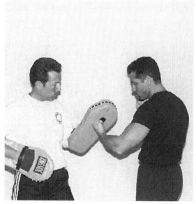

The rear shovel hook.

REAR SHOVEL HOOK

To properly execute the rear shovel hook, quickly dip your rear shoulder and simultaneously twist your rear leg and hip into your assailant's target; then drive your entire body into the assailant. Remember to always keep balanced.

Rear Shovel-Hook Training Exercise

The rear shovel hook can also be developed on either the heavy bag or the focus mitts. To begin, start from a right fighting stance and execute 25 powerful blows into the mitts. When you are done, switch to a left fighting stance and deliver 25 more.

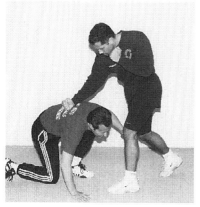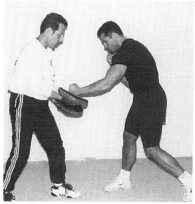

Rear vertical hammer fist (long arc).

REAR VERTICAL HAMMER FIST

The hammer fist (long arc) is a "finishing-off" technique that is delivered vertically to either the assailant's neck or spine. To deliver the rear vertical hammer fist, begin by raising your fist with your elbow flexed. Drive your clenched fist down in a vertical line onto the back of your assailant's neck. Be certain to bend at your hips and knees and follow through your target. Remember to keep your elbow bent on impact and maintain your balance throughout execution. **CAUTION:** *Never deliver a hammer-fist strike with a straight arm. This will rob you of speed and power and possibly cause a severe elbow strain.*

Rear Vertical Hammer-Fist Training Exercise

The focus mitts should be used for developing the vertical hammer fist. Start by having your training partner hold a pair of mitts at approximately waist level. Next, from a right fighting stance execute 15 powerful hammer fists into the mitts. Then switch your stance and deliver 15 more.

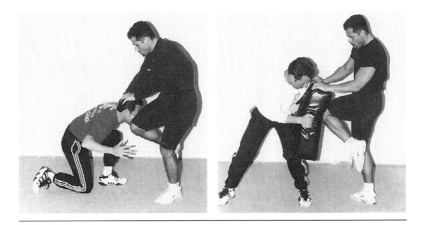

The rear vertical knee.

REAR VERTICAL KNEE

The rear vertical-knee strike is another devastating close-quarter grappling-range tool that can bring a formidable assailant to the ground. The knee strike travels vertically to a variety of anatomical targets, including the common peroneal nerve, the quadriceps, the groin, the ribs, and, in some cases, the face. When delivering the strike, be certain to make contact with your patella and not your lower thigh. To guarantee sufficient power, deliver all your knee strikes with your rear leg.

Rear Vertical-Knee Training Exercise

The rear vertical knee can be developed on the striking shield. Begin from a right fighting stance and launch 25 explosive strikes. Remember to take your time between each repetition. Switch your stance and deliver 25 more.

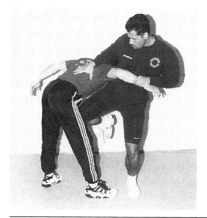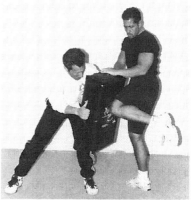

The rear diagonal knee.

REAR DIAGONAL KNEE

The rear diagonal-knee strike is another one that travels on a diagonal plane to the assailant, much like the hook kick. Targets include the common peroneal nerve, quadriceps, groin, ribs, and face. When delivering the strike, don't forget to follow through your target.

Rear Diagonal-Knee Training Exercise

The rear diagonal knee can also be developed on the kicking shield. Start by having your training partner hold the shield flush against his body. From a right fighting stance, deliver 25 accurate knee strikes into the shield. Switch your stance and deliver 25 more.

CONTINUAL PRACTICE IS ESSENTIAL

"Knowing" a technique is definitely not the same as being able to actually perform it—and performing a technique in a safe and secure training environment is not the same as being able to use it during a volatile street fight. Continual practice accompanied by realistic training scenarios is of the utmost importance. You must integrate the stressful and spontaneous elements of combat *safely* into your routine. This reality-based training is a sure-fire method of preparing you for the rigors of street fighting.

Keep in mind that the more acquainted you are with your first- and secondary-strike weapons, the more comfortable you'll be when deploying them against a formidable adversary. For example, a rear palm-heel strike will require thousands of repetitions for its employment to be embedded into your memory and allow you to use it reflexively, without conscious thought. The bottom line is this: If you are not willing to practice regularly, then don't ever expect these weapons to work for you in combat. The accompanying box shows a breakdown of the various weapons—don't ever forget them!

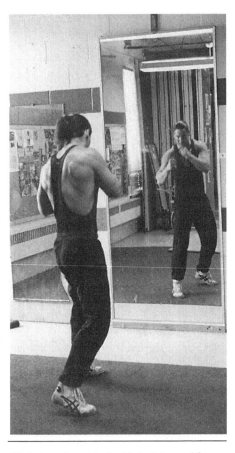

The mirror is an invaluable training tool for refining technique.

FIRST-STRIKE TOOLS
Vertical kick
Push kick
Finger jab
Rear palm heel
Rear vertical hammer fist (short arc)
Double-thumb gouge
Rear web-hand strike
Rear horizontal elbow
Rear diagonal elbow

ADVANCED FIRST-STRIKE TOOLS
Side kick
Horizontal hammer fist
Horizontal knife hand

SECONDARY-STRIKE TOOLS
Hook kick
Lead straight
Rear cross
Lead hook punch
Rear hook punch
Lead shovel-hook punch
Rear shovel-hook punch
Lead uppercut
Rear uppercut
Rear vertical hammer fist (long arc)
Rear vertical-knee strike
Rear diagonal-knee strike

TRAINING ROUTINES

The following training routines are designed to develop and refine both your first- and secondary-strike tools. Remember: *Repetition is the mother of skill.*

Beginner-Level Routine

Pace: Three-second pause between each repetition.
Vision: Eyes are open when executing each technique.

First-Strike Tools	Repetitions
Vertical kick	25
Push kick	25
Finger jab	50
Rear palm heel	25
Rear vertical hammer fist (short arc)	25
Double-thumb gouge	15
Web-hand strike	20
Rear horizontal elbow	25
Rear diagonal elbow	25

Advanced First-Strike Tools	Repetitions
Side kick	20
Horizontal hammer fist	20
Horizontal knife hand	20

Secondary-Strike Tools	Repetitions
Hook kick	25
Lead straight	25
Rear cross	25
Lead hook	25
Rear hook	25
Lead uppercut	25
Rear uppercut	25
Lead shovel hook	25
Rear shovel hook	25
Rear vertical hammer fist (long arc)	15

Rear vertical knee	25
Rear diagonal knee	25

Intermediate-Level Routine

Pace: One-second pause between each repetition.
Vision: Eyes are open when executing each technique.

First-Strike Tools	Repetitions
Vertical kick	75
Push kick	75
Finger jab	75
Rear palm heel	75
Rear vertical hammer fist (short arc)	75
Double-thumb gouge	75
Web-hand strike	75
Rear horizontal elbow	75
Rear diagonal elbow	75

Advanced First-Strike Tools	Repetitions
Side kick	50
Horizontal hammer fist	50

Secondary-Strike Tools	Repetitions
Hook kick	50
Lead straight	50
Rear cross	50
Lead hook	50
Rear hook	50
Lead uppercut	50
Rear uppercut	50
Lead shovel hook	50
Rear shovel hook	50
Rear vertical hammer fist (long arc)	50

Rear vertical knee	50
Rear diagonal knee	50

Advanced-Level Routine

Pace: No pause between each repetition.
Vision: Eyes are closed when executing each technique.

First-Strike Tools	Repetitions
Vertical kick	150–200
Push kick	150–200
Finger jab	150–200
Rear palm heel	150–200
Rear vertical hammer fist (short arc)	150–200
Double-thumb gouge	150–200
Web-hand strike	150–200
Rear horizontal elbow	150–200
Rear diagonal elbow	150–200

Advanced First-Strike Tools	Repetitions
Side kick	75–100
Horizontal hammer fist	75–100

Secondary-Strike Tools	Repetitions
Hook kick	100–175
Lead straight	100–175
Rear cross	100–175
Lead hook	100–175
Rear hook	100–175
Lead uppercut	100–175
Rear uppercut	100–175
Lead shovel hook	100–175
Rear shovel hook	100–175

Rear vertical hammer fist (long arc)   100–175
Rear vertical knee   100–175
Rear diagonal knee   100–175

CHAPTER 6

FIRST-STRIKE SCENARIOS

"I have come here to kick ass and chew bubble gum, and I'm all out of bubble gum."
—Roddy Piper

This chapter will illustrate 15 different first-strike scenarios. Because every street fight is unique, these scenarios only serve as examples of the possible combinations that can be deployed in combat. When reviewing and studying the photographs, pay particular attention to how I exploit my opponent's reaction dynamics.

SCENARIO 1

Vertical Kick/Rear Cross/Lead Hook/
Rear Hook/Rear Vertical Knee

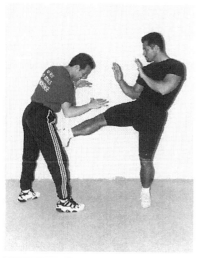 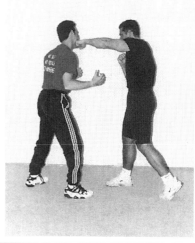

Sammy Franco is threatened at the kicking range of unarmed combat. From the first-strike stance, he employs disingenuous vocalization. Once the opponent is distracted, Franco attacks with a quick vertical kick.

Franco exploits his opponent's forward reaction dynamics by following up with a rear cross.

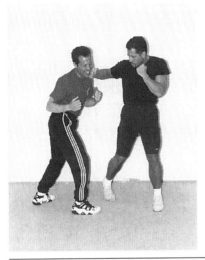

Franco then drives a lead hook to the temple . . .

. . . and follows with a rear hook to the head.

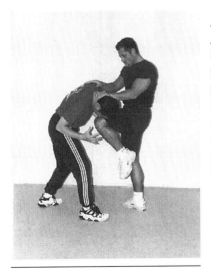

He then concludes his compound attack with a vertical knee strike.

FRANCO'S FIGHTING TIP

One of the most neglected aspects of a compound attack is proper breathing. Proper breathing promotes muscular relaxation, which increases the speed and efficiency of your compound attack. Remember to exhale whenever you deliver a blow.

FIRST STRIKE

Push Kick/Rear Uppercut/
Lead Horizontal Elbow/Rear Vertical Knee

FRANCO'S FIGHTING TIP
When employing punching-range techniques, don't forget to protect your face and chin with your shoulders.

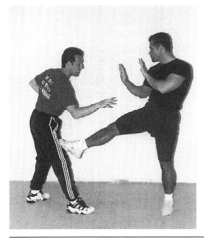
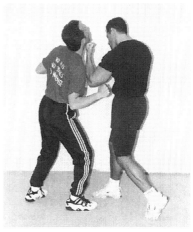

Sammy Franco is threatened at the kicking range of unarmed combat. He begins by employing disingenuous vocalization. Once his opponent is distracted, Franco attacks with a non telegraphic push kick.

Franco follows up with a rear uppercut to the chin.

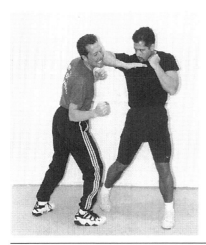
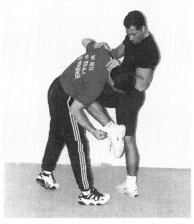

The lead horizontal elbow immediately follows.

The compound attack is concluded with a rear vertical-knee strike.

129

SCENARIO 3

Push Kick/Rear Cross

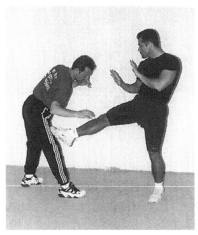 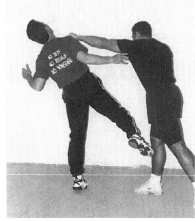

Franco assumes a first-strike stance and engages in disingenuous vocalization. Once the threatening opponent is distracted, Franco begins with an explosive push kick to his opponent's quadriceps (thigh).

Once the opponent drops his hand guard, Franco exploits the opening with an explosive rear cross. The rest is history!

FRANCO'S FIGHTING TIP

Because punching techniques constitute a large portion of your offensive arsenal, it's important to know how to make a proper fist. To make a fist, tightly clench the four fingers evenly in the palm of your hand and wrap your thumb securely over your index and middle fingers.

SCENARIO 4

Finger Jab/Rear Vertical Knee

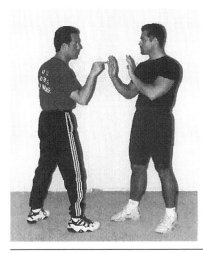

Franco assumes his first-strike stance.

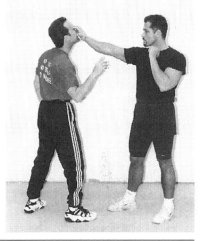

He wastes no time and attacks with a lightning-quick finger jab.

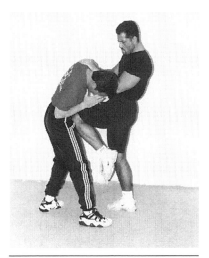

The opponent is neutralized with a rear vertical knee strike.

FRANCO'S FIGHTING TIP

Keep your wrists straight when executing punching techniques. If your wrist bends or collapses on impact, you will either sprain or break it, and that will take you out of the fight.

SCENARIO 5

Finger Jab/Rear Cross/Lead Straight/Rear Cross

FRANCO'S FIGHTING TIP

One very effective method of increasing the power of your linear punch is to step forward as you deliver your blow. Remember, this technique will only work if your punch is executed simultaneously as you step. Add this technique to your combat repertoire.

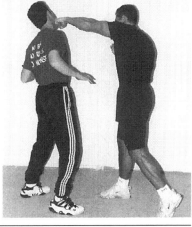

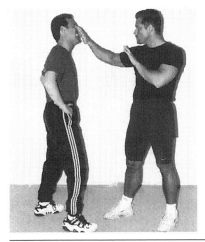

In this scenario, Franco launches his first strike from the punching range of unarmed combat. He begins with a lightning-quick finger-jab strike to the opponent's eyes.

Once the assailant's vision is impaired, Franco quickly follows up with a powerful rear cross to the face.

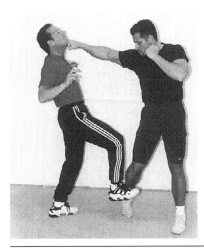

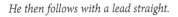

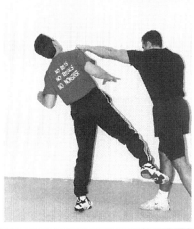

He then follows with a lead straight.

The compound attack is concluded with a final rear cross to the injured opponent.

FIRST STRIKE

SCENARIO 6

Finger Jab/Rear Palm Heel/Lead Hook/Rear Hook

FRANCO'S FIGHTING TIP

Americans are inveterate supporters of the underdog: they hate to see anyone lose a fight. Onlooker intervention is a common occurrence during a street fight. Therefore, when attacking your adversary, be cognizant of all spectators.

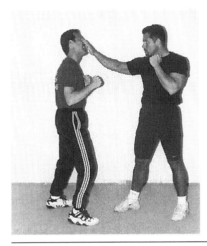

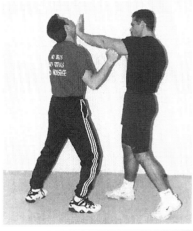

From the punching range, Franco employs disingenuous vocalization. At the ideal moment he attacks with a finger jab to the opponent's eyes.

Without a second's hesitation he follows with a rear palm-heel strike . . .

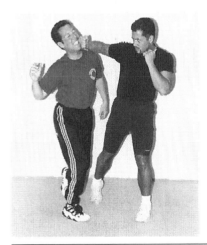

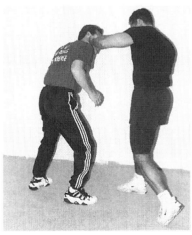

. . . and a lead hook.

The opponent is neutralized with a rear hook punch.

Rear Palm Heel/Lead Horizontal Elbow/ Rear Horizontal Elbow

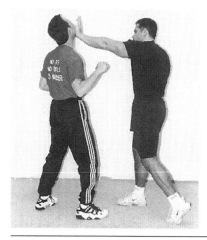

Franco launches a rear palm heel from his first-strike stance.

A lead horizontal elbow is now in order.

FRANCO'S FIGHTING TIP

There is nothing wrong with head-hunting in a street fight. Head-hunting means strategically selecting and pursuing the opponent's head as your primary impact target.

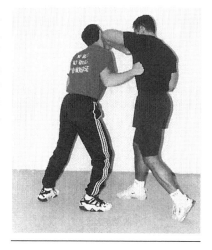

Franco moves in with a devastating rear horizontal elbow.

SCENARIO 8

Rear Palm Heel/Lead Shovel Hook/Rear Uppercut/Rear Vertical Knee

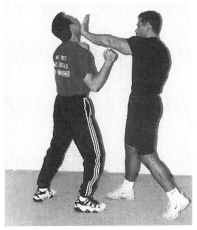 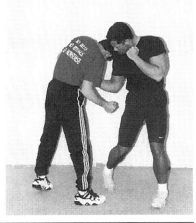

Franco is threatened by an opponent at the punching range of unarmed combat. From the first-strike stance, he employs disingenuous vocalization while simultaneously executing a rear palm heel to his assailant's chin.

He takes full advantage of the opponent's reaction dynamics by launching a lead shovel hook.

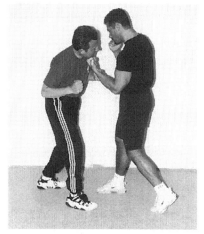

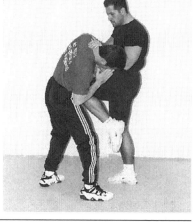

He immediately follows with a rear uppercut to the opponent's chin.

The compound attack is complete with a rear vertical-knee strike.

FRANCO'S FIGHTING TIP

The longer a street fight lasts, the greater your chances of serious injury or death. There is no time to design a battle plan or test the opponent's ability with probing techniques. Remember, a street fight should end as quickly as it begins.

SCENARIO 9

Rear Vertical Hammer Fist
(Short Arc)/Lead Hook/Rear Diagonal Knee

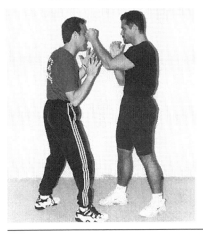 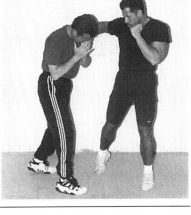

Franco is threatened in the grappling range of unarmed combat. From the grappling-range first-strike stance, he whips a rear vertical hammer fist against his opponent's nose.

Like a shark tasting blood, Franco immediately follows with a quick lead hook to the temple.

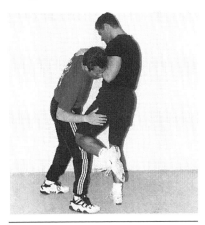

The opponent is finished off with a powerful rear diagonal-knee strike.

FRANCO'S FIGHTING TIP
Once the street fight is over and your opponent is neutralized, conduct an immediate inventory of yourself. Quickly scan your torso, hands, arms, legs, and feet for any sign of injury. Run your hands down your face, head, and neck to check for blood. If you are injured, get medical assistance immediately.

SCENARIO 10

Rear Vertical Hammer Fist (Short Arc)/Lead Horizontal Elbow/Rear Vertical Hammer Fist (Long Arc)

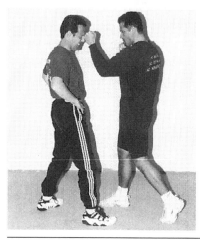 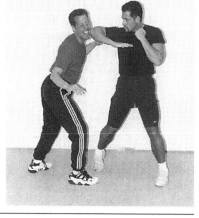

After engaging in disingenuous vocalization, Franco attacks his opponent with a rear vertical hammer fist (short arc).

Franco exploits the opponent's opening with a lead horizontal elbow.

FRANCO'S FIGHTING TIP
During the course of your compound attack, it's important to be mobile. When moving, remember to always move the foot that is closer to the direction you want to go first and then let the other foot follow at an equal distance. This prevents cross-stepping, which can be perilous.

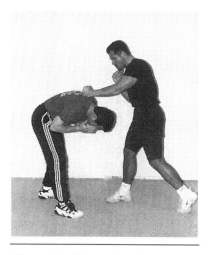

He completes his assault with a rear vertical hammer fist.

SCENARIO 11

Double-Thumb Gouge/Rear Vertical Knee/Rear Vertical Knee/Rear Vertical Hammer Fist (Long Arc)

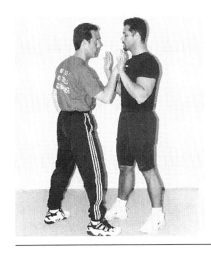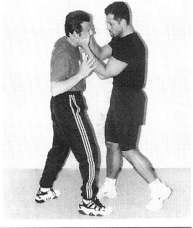

Franco is threatened at close quarters.

From the grappling-range first-strike stance, he employs disingenuous vocalization and immediately attacks with a double-thumb gouge.

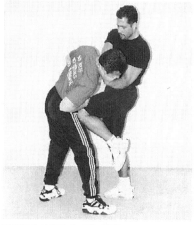

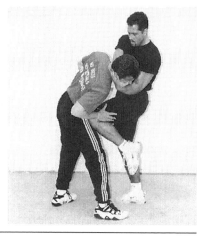

While maintaining the double-thumb gouge, Franco drives a rear vertical knee to his opponent's groin.

Franco keeps the pressure on with another vertical-knee strike.

FRANCO'S FIGHTING TIP

A well-seasoned street fighter can smell fear. If your adversary senses that you are frightened of him, it will reinforce his determination to destroy you in the street fight.

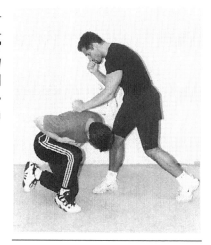

The compound attack is complete with a rear vertical hammer fist (long arc).

SCENARIO 12

Web-Hand Strike/Rear Diagonal Knee

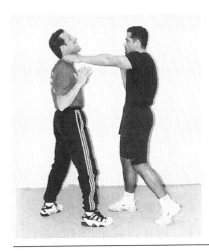 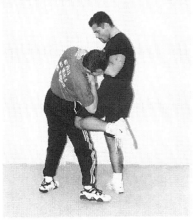

From the grappling range of unarmed combat, Franco executes a lightning-quick web-hand strike to his opponent's throat.

He ends it quickly with a diagonal-knee strike.

FRANCO'S FIGHTING TIP

After completing your compound attack, remember to "relocate" to the opponent's flank or flee the area completely.

SCENARIO 13

Rear Web-Hand Strike/Lead Diagonal Elbow/ Rear Vertical Knee

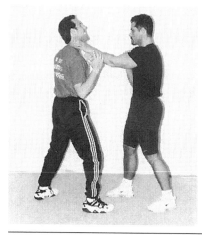

Franco attacks his opponent with a rear web-hand strike to the throat.

He then moves in with a lead diagonal-elbow strike.

FRANCO'S FIGHTING TIP
Although the first-strike principle is designed to give you a strategic blueprint for defeating a redoubtable opponent in a street fight, it's also vital that you possess the skill and ability to attack and defend spontaneously.

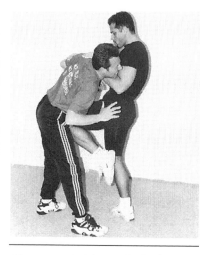

The rear vertical knee is the final weapon of choice.

SCENARIO 14

Rear Horizontal Elbow/Lead Horizontal Elbow/ Rear Diagonal Knee

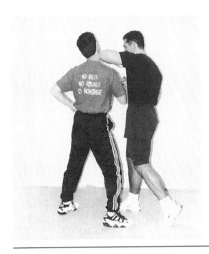 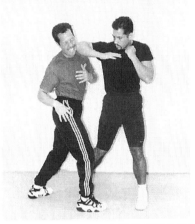

From the grappling-range first-strike stance, Franco delivers a rear horizontal elbow.

The opponent's reaction dynamics allow Franco to launch a lead horizontal elbow.

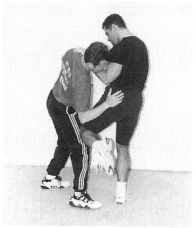

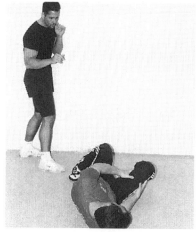

The threat is neutralized with a rear diagonal-knee strike.

Notice how Franco employs the relocation principle at the end of his compound attack.

FRANCO'S FIGHTING TIP

Be exceptionally accurate when delivering fisted blows at the opponent. One misplaced punch to the opponent's skull can easily break your hand and immediately put you out of commission.

SCENARIO 15

Rear Diagonal Elbow/Rear Vertical Knee/Rear Vertical Hammer Fist (Long Arc)

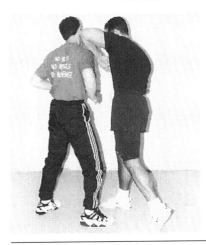

The first strike assault begins with a rear diagonal-elbow strike.

The opponent's reaction dynamics permit Franco to attack with a rear vertical knee.

FRANCO'S FIGHTING TIP

If you are going to precede your compound attack with a kick, be certain to bring your foot back to the ground as quickly as possible.

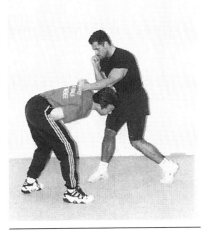

Franco puts his opponent out of his misery with a rear vertical hammer fist.

MULTIPLE-OPPONENT SCENARIOS

Defending against multiple opponents is a difficult and dangerous task. Although the odds are heavily against you, you can survive such a confrontation by employing some of the following advanced first-strike tools. What follows are some possible scenarios that you might encounter on the street.

ADVANCED SCENARIO 1

Vertical Hammer Fist (Short Arc)/Side Kick

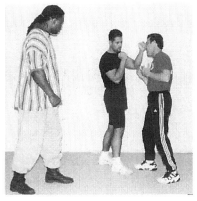
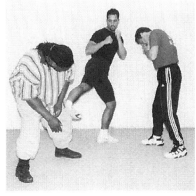

In this photo, Franco is confronted with multiple opponents. Without telegraphing his intentions, he delivers a vertical hammer fist (short arc) to the first opponent.

Franco moves in and attacks the second opponent with a side kick to the knee.

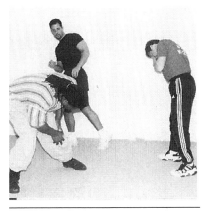

When the window of opportunity presents itself, Franco quickly escapes from the scene.

FRANCO'S FIGHTING TIP
Any physical action that does not directly contribute to your overall combat agenda is nothing more than an imprudent expenditure that can get you killed.

ADVANCED SCENARIO 2

Finger Jab/Horizontal Knife Hand

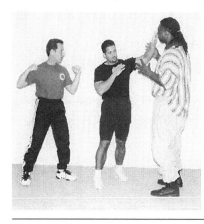 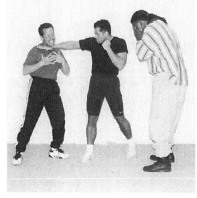

Franco is faced with two opponents. He launches a finger-jab strike to opponent number one . . .

. . . and immediately strikes opponent number two with a horizontal knife hand.

FRANCO'S FIGHTING TIP
Your head is the command center that controls the functioning of your entire body, and it's the most important target to protect in a street fight. By maintaining a proper fighting stance and keeping your chin angled down, you will help keep it out of harm's way.

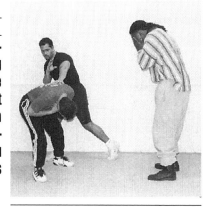

Franco then escapes to safety.

MAKESHIFT-WEAPON SCENARIO

A makeshift weapon can be used to deliver a first strike. Makeshift weapons are common, everyday objects that can be converted into either offensive or defensive weapons. (For more information about makeshift weapons, see *When Seconds Count*.) The following scenario is just one example of a first-strike makeshift weapon.

Briefcase/Hook Kick/Rear Hook Punch

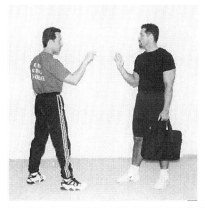 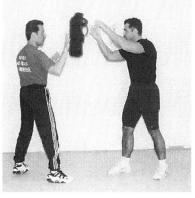

Franco is threatened by an opponent.

He throws his briefcase at his opponent's face.

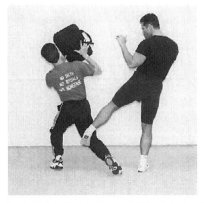 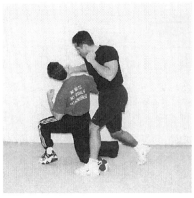

He then exploits his assailant's reaction dynamics with a powerful hook kick . . .

. . . and follows with a rear hook punch.

KNOW HOW TO DEAL WITH THE POLICE

After a street fight, there is always the possibility that you will have to deal with the police. Keep in mind that a police officer is permitted to approach you in a public place and request information. Furthermore, if the officer reasonably suspects that you are committing, have committed, or are about to commit a crime, he may detain you briefly for questioning.

If a police officer reasonably suspects that you are armed and dangerous, he is permitted to frisk you without making an arrest. If while frisking you for weapons or evidence, the officer finds anything illegal, he can confiscate it and arrest you. What follows are seven simple rules of conduct when confronted by an officer of the law.

1. *Identify yourself as the victim.* Be prepared to show identification, but be careful to avoid quick or sudden movements when reaching for your wallet and always try to keep your hands in plain view.
2. *Be polite and respectful to the officer.* Don't talk back and always address him or her as either "sir" or "ma'am."
3. *Watch what you say.* Speak slowly and clearly, avoid using profanity, sarcasm, and racial or derogatory remarks, and realize

that what you say can be used against you.

4. *Explain what happened.* Clearly describe the sequence of events that led to the fight and whether the assailant used a weapon.

5. *Follow orders.* If the officer orders you to wait at a particular spot while he sorts out the matter, obey him.

6. *Don't get angry.* If you get angry or hostile with police officers, you will land in jail.

7. *Know your rights.* Finally, if you are arrested and taken into police custody, remember that you have the right to remain silent, obtain a lawyer, be informed of the charges against you, and have a judge decide whether you should be released on bail.

DISINGENUOUS VOCALIZATION EXERCISES

Both the Gemini principle and the fifth-column tactic are terrific combat strategies that are not easily mastered. Many hours must be devoted to developing and refining the ability to speak calmly and strike simultaneously. Here are four effective vocalization exercises that will help you develop this deceptive and indispensable skill.

PLEDGE DRILL

This exercise requires that you verbally recite the pledge of allegiance. While you are reciting the pledge your training partner is to yell, "Attack!" and you are to immediately launch a preselected compound attack in the air. The key is to deliver a flurry of full-speed, full-force strikes *while continuing* to recite the pledge in a calm and controlled manner. It's critical that you do not alter the tone, pitch, volume, or tempo of your voice when delivering your assault.

NURSERY RHYME DRILL
(BEGINNER LEVEL)

This exercise is similar to "the pledge" except that it requires you to verbally recite a simple children's nursery rhyme, such as "Mary Had a Little Lamb" or "Hickory, Dickory, Dock." Once again, while you are reciting the rhyme, your training partner yells, "Attack!" and you are to immediately launch a preselected compound attack in the air without disturbing the vocalization of the rhyme. Once again, it's critical not to alter the tonality of your voice when delivering your assault.

TONGUE TWISTER
(INTERMEDIATE LEVEL)

The tongue twister is an intermediate-level drill that requires you to slowly and repeatedly recite a tongue twister, such as "She sells seashells on the seashore of Seychelles" or "Peter Piper picked a peck of pickled peppers." While you are reciting this statement, your training partner is to yell, "Attack!" and you must immediately launch a preselected compound attack in the air. Once again, it's critical that you do not disturb the vocalization or alter the tone, pitch, volume, or tempo of your voice when delivering your assault.

THE ALPHABET
(ADVANCED LEVEL)

The "alphabet" is a more advanced drill. Your objective here is to slowly recite the alphabet *backward*. At some point during your recitation, your training partner is to yell, "Attack!" and you are to immediately launch a preselected compound attack in the air while continuing to recite the alphabet backwards. Don't get frustrated with this exercise; it's designed to challenge you.

SAMPLE COMPOUND ATTACKS

What follows are five sample compound attacks that can be employed when conducting the vocalization exercises. (For more compound attacks, please see Chapter 6.)

When executing your attack, make certain your strikes are delivered with speed, power, and proper form. Also keep in mind that you can practice in front of a mirror, on the heavy bag, or on the focus mitts.

1. Push kick/finger jab/rear vertical hammer fist (long arc)
2. Vertical kick/rear cross/lead horizontal elbow/rear horizontal elbow
3. Finger jab/rear cross/lead straight/rear cross
4. Rear palm heel/rear vertical hammer fist/rear vertical knee
5. Rear horizontal elbow/lead horizontal elbow/rear horizontal elbow

GLOSSARY

The following terms are defined in the context of Contemporary Fighting Arts and its related concepts. In some instances, the definitions bear little resemblance to those found in a standard dictionary.

accuracy—The precise or exact projection of force. Accuracy is also defined as the ability to execute a combat movement with precision and exactness.

adaptability—The ability to adjust physically and psychologically to new or different conditions or circumstances of combat.

adrenaline dump—The process of adrenaline (epinephrine) being rapidly released into your bloodstream in response to a fighting situation.

advanced first-strike tools—Offensive techniques specifically used to initiate a first strike against multiple opponents.

aerobic exercise—"With air." Exercise that elevates the heart rate to a training level for a prolonged period, usually 30 minutes.

aggression—Hostile and injurious behavior directed toward a person.

aggressive hand positioning—Placement of the hands so as to imply aggressive or hostile intentions.

agility—An attribute of combat. One's ability to move one's body quickly and gracefully.

ambidextrous—The ability to perform with equal facility on both the right and left sides of the body.

analysis and integration—One of the five elements of CFA's mental component. This is the painstaking process of breaking down various elements, concepts, sciences, and disciplines into their constituent parts, and then methodically and strategically analyzing, experimenting, and drastically modifying the information so that it fulfills three combat requirements: efficiency, effectiveness, and safety. Only then is it finally integrated into the CFA system.

anatomical striking targets—The various body targets that can be struck and that are especially vulnerable to potential harm. They include the eyes, temple, nose, chin, back of neck, front of neck, solar plexus, ribs, groin, thighs, knees, shins, and instep.

assailant—A person who threatens or attacks another person.

assault—The willful attempt or threat to inflict injury upon the person of another.

assault and battery—The unlawful touching of another person without justification.

assessment—The process of rapidly and accurately gathering, analyzing, and evaluating information in terms of threat and danger. You can assess people, places, actions, and objects.

attack—Offensive action designed to physically control, injure, or kill another person.

attributes of combat—The physical, mental, and spiritual qualities that enhance combat skills and tactics.

awareness—Perception or knowledge of people, places, actions, and objects. (For the purposes of this book there are three categories of tactical awareness: criminal, situational, and self-awareness.)

B

balance—One's ability to maintain equilibrium while stationary or moving.

ballistics—The study of the firing, flight, and effects of ammunition.

barriers—Any object that obstructs the enemy's path of attack.

blading the body—Strategically positioning your body at a 45-degree angle.

block—A defensive tool designed to intercept the assailant's attack by placing a nonvital target between the assailant's strike and your vital body target.

body composition—The ratio of fat to lean body tissue.

body language—Nonverbal communication through posture, gestures, and facial expressions.

body mechanics—Technically precise body movement during the execution of a body weapon, defensive technique, or other fighting maneuver.

body weapon—One of the various body parts that can be used to strike or otherwise injure or kill a criminal assailant. (Also known as tool.)

C

cadence—Coordinating tempo and rhythm to establish a timing pattern of movement.

cardiorespiratory conditioning—The component of physical fitness that deals with the heart, lungs, and circulatory system.

centerline—An imaginary vertical line that divides your body in half and contains many of your vital anatomical targets.

circular movement—Movements that follow the direction of a curve.

close-quarter combat—One of the three ranges of knife and bludgeon combat. At this distance, you can strike, slash, or stab your assailant with a variety of close-quarter techniques.

cognitive development—One of the five elements of CFA's mental component. The process of developing and enhancing your fighting skills through specific mental exercises and techniques. (See *analysis and integration, killer instinct, philosophy,* and *strategic/tactical development.*)

cognitive exercises—Various mental exercises used to enhance fighting skills and tactics.

combat arts—The various arts of war.

combat attributes—(See *attributes of combat.*)

combat fitness—A state characterized by cardiorespiratory and muscular/skeletal conditioning, as well as proper body composition.

combat mentality—A combative state of mind necessary for fighting. Also known as the killer instinct. (See *killer instinct.*)

combat ranges—The various ranges of unarmed combat.

combat utility—The quality or condition of being useful in combat.

combination(s)—(See *compound attack.*)

common peroneal nerve—A pressure point area located approximately four to six inches above the knee on the midline of the outside of the thigh.

composure—A combat attribute. Composure is a quiet and focused mind-set that enables you to achieve your combat agenda.

compound attack—One of the five conventional methods of attack. Two or more body weapons launched in strategic succession whereby the fighter overwhelms his assailant with a flurry of full-speed, full-force blows.

conditioning training—A training methodology requiring the practitioner to deliver a variety of offensive and defensive combinations for a four-minute period. (See *proficiency training* and *street training.*)

Contemporary Fighting Arts (CFA)—A modern martial art and self-defense system made up of three parts: physical, mental, and spiritual.

conventional ground fighting tools—Specific ground fighting techniques designed to control, restrain, and temporarily incapacitate your adversary. Some conventional ground fighting tactics include submission holds, locks, certain choking techniques, and specific striking techniques.

coordination—A physical attribute characterized by the ability to perform a technique or movement with efficiency, balance, and accuracy.

counterattack—Offensive action made to counter an assailant's initial attack.

courage—A combat attribute. The state of mind and spirit that enables a fighter to face danger and vicissitudes with confidence, resolution, and bravery.

courageousness—(See *courage.*)

criminal awareness—One of the three categories of CFA awareness. It involves a general understanding and knowledge of the nature and dynamics of a criminal's motivations, mentalities, methods, and capabilities to perpetrate violent crime. (See *situational awareness* and *self-awareness.*)

criminal justice—The study of criminal law and the procedures associated with its enforcement.

criminology—The scientific study of crime and criminals.

cross-stepping—The process of crossing one foot in front or behind the other when moving.

crushing tactics—Nuclear grappling-range techniques designed to crush the assailant's anatomical targets.

D

deadly force—Weapons or techniques that may result in imminent unconsciousness, permanent disfigurement, or death.

deception—A combat attribute. A stratagem whereby you delude your assailant.

decisiveness—A combat attribute. The ability to follow a tactical course of action that is unwavering and focused.

defense—The ability to strategically thwart an assailant's attack (armed or unarmed).

defensive execution—The third and final stage of defensive reaction time wherein your body executes the appropriate defensive response.

defensive fighter—One who permits his adversary to seize and maintain offensive control in a fight.

defensive flow—A progression of continuous defensive responses.

defensive mentality—A defensive mind-set.

defensive reaction time—The elapsed time between the assailant's physical attack (e.g., punch, kick, throat grab) and your defensive response to that attack (e.g., block, parry, evasion movement). Defensive reaction time is the result of three stages (defensive recognition, defensive selection, and defensive execution).

defensive recognition—The first stage of defensive reaction time where you realize and identify that an attack has occurred.

defensive selection—The second stage of defensive reaction time wherein you immediately select the appropriate defensive response.

demeanor—One of the essential factors to consider when assessing a threatening individual. A person's outward behavior.

diet—A lifestyle of healthy eating.

disingenuous vocalization—See *Gemini principle.*

distancing—The ability to quickly understand spatial relationships and how they relate to combat.

distractionary tactics—Various verbal and physical tactics designed to distract your adversary.

E

effectiveness—One of the three criteria for a body weapon, technique, tactic, or maneuver. It means the ability to produce a desired effect. (See *efficiency* and *safety.*)

efficiency—One of the three criteria for a body weapon, technique, tactic, or maneuver. It means the ability to reach an objective quickly and economically. (See *effectiveness* and *safety.*)

elbow block—An arm block used to stop circular blows aimed at your head or upper torso.

emotionless—A combat attribute. Being temporarily devoid of human feeling.

escape routes—The various avenues or exits that allow you to safely flee from a threatening situation.

evasion—A defensive maneuver that allows you to strategically maneuver your body away from an assailant's strike.

evasive sidestepping—Evasive footwork where the practitioner moves to either the right or left side.

evasiveness—A combat attribute. The ability to avoid threat or danger.

excessive force—An amount of force that exceeds the need for a particular event and is unjustified in the eyes of the law.

experimentation—The painstaking process of testing a combat hypothesis or theory.

explosiveness—A combat attribute that is characterized by a sudden outburst of violent energy.

fear—A strong and unpleasant emotion caused by the anticipation or awareness of threat or danger. There are three stages of fear (in order of intensity): fright, panic, and terror. (See *fright, panic, terror.*)

fear management—The ability to manage and control the deleterious effects of fear.

femoral nerve—A pressure point area located approximately six inches above the knee on the inside of the thigh.

fifth-column tactic—A first-strike tactic used when a significant other (e.g., close friend, spouse, acquaintance, co-worker, partner) is threatened by an assailant. The fifth-column tactic is the strategic and deceptive use of both verbal and nonverbal skills that enable you to effectively launch a first strike at your enemy.

fighting stance—One of the different types of stances used in this book. A strategic posture you can assume when face-to-face with an unarmed assailant. The fighting stance is used after you have launched your first-strike tool.

fight-or-flight syndrome—A response of the sympathetic nervous system to a fearful and threatening situation, during which it prepares your body to either fight or flee from the perceived danger.

finesse—A combat attribute. The ability to skillfully execute a movement or a series of movements with grace and refinement.

first strike—The strategic application of proactive force designed to interrupt the initial stages of an assault before it becomes a self-defense situation.

first-strike prerequisites—The 11 requirements necessary to safely and effectively launch a first strike in a self-defense situation. These prerequisites include range proficiency, stances, mobility, body weapon mastery, target awareness, combat attributes, compound attack and the offensive flow, "Gemini" principle, fifth-column tactic, fear management, and the killer instinct.

first-strike principle—A principle that states that when physical danger is imminent and you have no other tactical option but to fight back, you should strike first, strike fast, and strike with authority and keep the pressure on.

first-strike stance—One of the different types of stances used in this book. A strategic posture used prior to initiating a first strike.

first-strike tools—Offensive tools specifically designed to initiate a preemptive strike against your adversary.

flexibility—The muscles' ability to move through maximum natural ranges. (See *muscular/skeletal conditioning.*)

footwork—Quick, economical steps performed on the balls of the feet while you are relaxed, alert, and balanced. Footwork is structured around four general movements: forward, backward, right, and left.

fractal tool—Offensive or defensive tools that can be used in more than one combat range.

fright—The first stage of fear; quick and sudden fear. (See *panic* and *terror.*)

G

Gemini principle—The Gemini principle is the strategic and deceptive use of both verbal and nonverbal skills that enables you to effectively launch a first strike at your enemy.

ghosting—The strategic process of mentally eliminating facial features on your adversary so that he appears faceless. Ghosting is most commonly used to prevent staring and for pseudospeciation enhancement.

grappling range—One of the three ranges of unarmed combat. Grappling range is the closest distance of unarmed combat from which you can employ a wide variety of close-quarter tools and techniques. The grappling range of unarmed combat is also divided into two different planes: vertical (standing) and horizontal (ground fighting). (See *kicking range* and *punching range.*)

grappling-range tools—The various body tools and techniques that are employed in the grappling range of unarmed combat, including head butts; biting, tearing, clawing, crushing, and gouging tactics; foot stomps; horizontal, vertical, and diagonal elbow strikes; vertical and diagonal knee strikes; chokes; strangles; joint locks; and holds. (See *kicking-range tools* and *punching-range tools*.)

ground fighting—Fighting that takes place on the ground. (Also known as horizontal grappling plane.)

guard—A fighter's hand positioning.

hand positioning—(See *guard*.)

head hunting—Strategically selecting and pursuing the opponent's head as a primary impact target.

heavy bag—A large cylindrical-shaped bag that is used to develop kicking, punching, or striking power.

high block—An arm block used to defend against overhead blows aimed at your head.

high-line kick—One of the two different classifications of kicks. A kick that is directed to targets above an assailant's waist level. (See *low-line kick*.)

histrionics—The field of theatrics or acting.

hook kick—A circular kick that can be delivered in both kicking and punching ranges.

hook punch—A circular punch that can be delivered in both the punching and grappling ranges.

impact power—Destructive force generated by mass and velocity.

impact training—A training exercise that develops pain tolerance.

incapacitate—To disable an assailant by rendering him unconscious or damaging his bones, joints, or organs.

initiative—Making the first offensive move in combat.

intent—One of the essential factors to consider when assessing a threatening individual. The assailant's purpose or motive. (See *demeanor, positioning, range,* and *weapon capability.*)

intuition—The innate ability to know or sense something without the use of rational thought.

invisible deployment—(See *non telegraphic movement.*)

joint lock—A grappling-range technique that immobilizes the assailant's joint.

K

kick—A sudden, forceful strike with the foot.

kicking range—One of the three ranges of unarmed combat. Kicking range is the farthest distance of unarmed combat wherein you can use your legs to strike an assailant. (See *grappling range* and *punching range.*)

kicking-range tools—The various body weapons employed in the kicking range of unarmed combat, including side kicks, push kicks, hook kicks, and vertical kicks.

killer instinct—A cold, primal mentality that surges to your consciousness and turns you into a vicious fighter.

kinesics—The study of nonlinguistic body movement communications (e.g., eye movement, shrugs, facial gestures).

kinesiology—The study of the principles and mechanics of human movement.

kinesthetic perception—The ability to accurately feel your body during the execution of a particular movement.

L

lead side—The side of the body that faces an assailant.

lethal force—The amount of force that can cause serious bodily injury or death.

linear movement—Movements that follow the path of a straight line.

lock—(See *joint lock*.)

low-line kick—One of the two different classifications of a kick. A kick that is directed to targets below the assailant's waist level. (See *high-line kick*.)

low-maintenance tool—An offensive and defensive tool that requires the least amount of training and practice to maintain proficiency. Low-maintenance tools generally don't require preliminary stretching.

makeshift weapon—A common everyday object that can be converted into either an offensive or defensive weapon. Some makeshift weapons can be used to deliver a first strike.

maneuver—To manipulate into a strategically desired position.

mechanics—(See *body mechanics.*)

mental attributes—The various cognitive qualities that enhance your fighting skills.

mental component—One of the three vital components of the CFA system. The mental component comprises the cerebral aspects of fighting, including the killer instinct, strategic and tactical development, analysis and integration, philosophy, and cognitive development. (See *physical component* and *spiritual component.*)

mental speed—The rate at which you can think and employ various cognitive skills in a combat situation.

mid-block—An arm block used to defend against circular blows aimed at your head or upper torso.

mobility—A combat attribute. The ability to move your body quickly and freely while balanced. (See *footwork.*)

modern martial art—A pragmatic combat art that has evolved to meet the demands and characteristics of the present time.

muscular endurance—The muscles' ability to perform the same motion or task repeatedly for a prolonged period.

muscular flexibility—The muscles' ability to move through maximum natural ranges.

muscular strength—The maximum force that can be exerted by a particular muscle or muscle group against resistance.

muscular/skeletal conditioning—An element of physical fitness that entails muscular strength, endurance, and flexibility.

neutralize—(See *incapacitate.*)

neutral zone—The distance outside of the kicking range from which neither the practitioner nor the assailant can touch each other.

nonaggressive physiology—Strategic body language used prior to initiating a first strike.

nonlethal force—The amount of force that does not cause serious bodily injury or death.

non-telegraphic movement—Body mechanics or movements that do not inform an assailant of your intentions. Also known as invisible deployment.

nuclear ground-fighting tools—Specific grappling-range tools designed to inflict immediate and irreversible damage. Some nuclear tools and tactics are biting tactics, tearing tactics, crushing tactics, continuous choking tactics, gouging techniques, raking tactics, and all striking techniques.

offense—The armed and unarmed means and methods of attacking a criminal assailant.

offensive flow—A progression of continuous offensive movements or actions designed to neutralize or terminate your adversary. (See *compound attack*.)

offensive reaction time—The elapsed time between offensive recognition and offensive execution.

one-mindedness—A state of deep concentration wherein you are free from all distractions (internal and external).

1,000-yard stare—One of the nonverbal signs that violence is possible. The 1,000-yard stare is when the adversary looks right through you.

ostrich defense—One common response of a frightened fighter. The practitioner will look away from that which he fears (e.g., punches, kicks, and strikes). The thinking of a person who employs this defense is, "*If I can't see it, it can't hurt me.*"

pain tolerance—Your ability to physically and psychologically withstand pain.

panic—The second stage of fear; overpowering fear. (See *fright* and *terror*.)

parry—A defensive technique; a quick, forceful slap that redirects an assailant's linear attack.

patience—A combat attribute. The ability to endure and tolerate difficulty.

perception—Interpretation of vital information acquired from your senses when faced with a potentially threatening situation.

philosophical resolution—The act of analyzing and answering various questions concerning the use of violence in defense of yourself and others.

philosophy—One of the five aspects of CFA's mental component. A deep state of introspection whereby you methodically resolve critical questions concerning the use of force in defense of yourself or others.

physical attributes—The numerous physical qualities that enhance your combat skills and abilities.

physical component—One of the three vital components of the CFA system. The physical component comprises the physical aspects of fighting, including physical fitness, weapon/technique mastery, and combat attributes. (See *mental component* and *spiritual component*.)

physical conditioning—(See *combat fitness*.)

physical fitness—(See *combat fitness*.)

physiognomy—The art of judging human character from facial features.

positioning—The spatial relationship of the assailant to his victim in terms of target exposure, escape, angle of attack, and various other strategic considerations.

positions of concealment—Various locations or objects that allow you to hide from your enemy temporarily.

post-traumatic syndrome—A group of symptoms that may occur in the aftermath of a violent confrontation with a criminal assailant. Common symptoms of post-traumatic syndrome include denial, shock, fear, anger, severe depression, sleeping and eating disorders, societal withdrawal, and paranoia.

power—A physical attribute of armed and unarmed combat. The amount of force you can generate when striking an anatomical target.

precision—(See *accuracy*.)

preemptive strike—(See *first strike*.)

premise—An axiom, concept, rule, or any other valid reason to modify or go beyond that which has been established.

proficiency training—A training methodology requiring the practitioner to execute a specific body weapon, technique, maneuver, or tactic over and over for a prescribed number or repetitions. (See *conditioning training* and *street training*.)

proxemics—The study of the nature and effect of man's personal space.

proximity—The ability to maintain a strategically safe distance from a threatening individual.

pseudospeciation—A combat attribute. The tendency to assign sub-human and inferior qualities to a threatening assailant.

psychological conditioning—The process of conditioning the mind for the horrors and rigors of real combat.

psychomotor speed—The rate at which you can move your body (e.g., punching, blocking, evading) in a street fighting situation.

punch—A quick, forceful strike of the fist.

punching range—One of the three ranges of unarmed combat. Punching range is the midrange of unarmed combat from which the fighter uses his hands to strike his assailant. (See *kicking range* and *grappling range*.)

punching-range tools—The various body weapons that are employed in the punching range of unarmed combat, including finger jabs, palm-heel strikes, rear cross, knife-hand strikes, horizontal and shovel hooks, uppercuts, and hammer-fist strikes. (See *grappling-range tools* and *kicking-range tools*.)

qualities of combat—(See *attributes of combat*.)

range—The spatial relationship between a fighter and a threatening assailant.

range deficiency—The inability to effectively fight and defend in all ranges (armed and unarmed) of combat.

range manipulation—A combat attribute. The strategic manipulation of combat ranges.

range proficiency—A combat attribute. The ability to effectively fight and defend in all ranges (armed and unarmed) of combat.

ranges of engagement—(See *combat ranges.*)

ranges of unarmed combat—The three distances in which a fighter might physically engage with an assailant while involved in unarmed combat: kicking, punching, and grappling.

reaction dynamics—The assailant's physical response to a particular tool, technique, or weapon after initial contact is made.

reaction time—The elapsed time between a stimulus and the response to that particular stimulus. (See *offensive reaction time* and *defensive reaction time.*)

rear cross—A straight punch delivered from the rear hand that crosses from right to left (if in a left stance) or left to right (if in a right stance).

rear side—The side of the body farthest from the assailant. (See *lead side.*)

reasonable force—That degree of force that is not excessive for a particular event and is appropriate for protecting yourself or others.

recovery breathing—The active process of quickly restoring your breathing to its normal state.

refinement—The strategic and methodical process of improving or perfecting.

relocating—A street fighting tactic that requires you to immediately move to a new location (usually by flanking your adversary) after delivering a compound attack.

repetition—Performing a single movement, exercise, strike, or action continuously for a specific period.

research—A scientific investigation or inquiry.

rhythm—Movement characterized by the natural ebb and flow of related elements.

S

safety—One of the three criteria for a body weapon, technique, maneuver, or tactic. It means that the tool, technique, maneuver, or tactic provides the least amount of danger and risk for the practitioner. (See *effectiveness* and *efficiency*.)

secondary-strike tools—Offensive techniques that are employed immediately after a first strike is launched.

self-awareness—One of the three categories of awareness. Knowing and understanding yourself. This includes aspects of yourself that may provoke criminal violence and that will promote a proper and strong reaction to an attack. (See *criminal awareness* and *situational awareness*.)

self-confidence—Having trust and faith in yourself.

self-enlightenment—The state of knowing your capabilities, limitations, character traits, feelings, general attributes, and motivations. (See *self-awareness*.)

set—A term used to describe a grouping of repetitions.

shadow fighting—A training exercise used to develop and refine your tools, techniques, and attributes of armed and unarmed combat.

single attack—(Also known as simple attack.) A method of attack whereby the fighter delivers a solitary offensive strike. It may involve a series of discrete probes or one swift and powerful strike aimed at terminating the fight.

situational awareness—One of the three categories of awareness. A state of being totally alert to your immediate surroundings, including people, places, objects, and actions. (See *criminal awareness* and *self-awareness*.)

skeletal alignment—The proper alignment or arrangement of your body. Skeletal alignment maximizes the structural integrity of striking tools.

slipping—A defensive maneuver that permits you to avoid an assailant's linear blow without stepping out of range. Slipping can be accomplished by quickly snapping the head and upper torso sideways (right or left) to avoid the blow.

snap back—A defensive maneuver that permits you to avoid an assailant's linear and circular blow without stepping out of range. The snap back can be accomplished by quickly snapping the head backward to avoid the assailant's blow.

speed—A physical and mental attribute of armed and unarmed combat. The rate or measure of the rapid rate of motion or thought process. There are two types of speed: mental and psychomotor.

spiritual component—One of the three vital components of the CFA system. The spiritual component comprises the metaphysical issues and aspects of existence. (See *physical component* and *mental component*.)

square off—To be face-to-face with a hostile or threatening assailant who is about to attack you.

stance—One of the many strategic postures that you assume before or during armed or unarmed combat.

strategic positioning—Tactically positioning yourself to either escape, move behind a barrier, or use a makeshift weapon.

strategy—A carefully planned method of achieving your goal of engaging an assailant under advantageous conditions.

street fight—A spontaneous and violent confrontation between two or more individuals wherein *no* rules apply.

street fighter—An unorthodox combatant who has no formal training. His combative skills and tactics are usually developed in the street by the process of trial and error.

street training—A training methodology requiring the practitioner to deliver explosive compound attacks for 10 to 20 seconds. (See *conditioning training* and *proficiency training*.)

strength training—The process of developing muscular strength through systematic application of progressive resistance.

striking art—A combat art that relies predominantly on striking techniques to neutralize or terminate a criminal attacker.

striking shield—A rectangular-shaped shield constructed of foam and vinyl used to develop power in most of your kicks, punches, and strikes.

striking tool—A natural body weapon that is used to hit the assailant's anatomical target.

strong side—The strongest and most coordinated side of your body.

structure—A definite and organized pattern.

style—The distinct manner in which a fighter executes or performs his combat skills.

stylistic integration—The purposeful and scientific collection of tools and techniques from various disciplines that are strategically integrated and dramatically altered to meet three essential criteria: efficiency, effectiveness, and combat safety.

system—The unification of principles, philosophies, rules, strategies, methodologies, tools, and techniques or a particular method of combat.

T

tactic—The skill of using the available means to achieve an end.

target awareness—A combat attribute that encompasses five strategic principles: target orientation, target recognition, target selection, target impact, and target exploitation.

target exploitation—A combat attribute. The strategic maximization of your assailant's reaction dynamics during a fight. Target exploitation can be applied in both armed and unarmed encounters.

target impact—The successful striking of the appropriate anatomical target.

target orientation—A combat attribute. Having a workable knowledge of the assailant's anatomical targets.

target recognition—The ability to immediately recognize appropriate anatomical targets during an emergency self-defense situation.

target selection—The process of mentally selecting the appropriate anatomical target for your self-defense situation. This is predicated on certain factors, including proper force response, assailant's positioning, and range.

target stare—A form of telegraphing whereby you stare at the anatomical target you intend to strike.

target zones—The three areas in which an assailant's anatomical targets are located. (See *zone one, zone two,* and *zone three.*)

technique—A systematic procedure by which a task is accomplished.

telegraphic cognizance—A combat attribute. The ability to recognize both verbal and nonverbal signs of aggression or assault.

telegraphing—Unintentionally making your intentions known to your adversary.

tempo—The speed or rate at which you speak.

terminate—The act of killing.

terror—The third stage of fear; defined as overpowering fear. (See *fright* and *panic.*)

timing—A physical and mental attribute of armed and unarmed combat. Your ability to execute a movement at the precise moment.

tone—The overall quality or character of your voice.

tool—(See *body weapon.*)

training drills—The various exercises and drills aimed at perfecting combat skills, attributes, and tactics.

unified mind—A mind that is free and clear of distractions and focused on the combat situation.

use-of-force response—A combat attribute. Selecting the appropriate level of force for a particular emergency self-defense situation.

viciousness—A combat attribute. Dangerously aggressive behavior.

violence—The intentional use of physical force to coerce, injure, cripple, or kill.

visualization—The purposeful formation of mental images and scenarios in the mind's eye.

warm-up—A series of mild exercises, stretches, and movements designed to prepare you for more intense exercise.

weak side—The weaker and more uncoordinated side of your body.

weapon and technique mastery—An element of CFA's physical component. The kinesthetic and psychomotor development of a weapon or combat technique.

weapon capability—An assailant's ability to use and attack with a particular weapon.

yell—A loud and aggressive scream or shout used for various strategic reasons.

Z

zone one—Anatomical targets related to your senses, including the eyes, temple, nose, chin, and back of neck.

zone three—Anatomical targets related to your mobility, including thighs, knees, shins, and instep.

zone two—Anatomical targets related to your breathing, including front of neck, solar plexus, ribs, and groin.

ABOUT THE AUTHOR

Sammy Franco is one of the world's foremost authorities on armed and unarmed combat. Highly regarded as a leading innovator in close-quarters combat, Mr. Franco was one of the premier pioneers in the field of "reality-based" self-defense instruction.

Convinced of the limited usefulness of martial arts in real street fighting situations, Mr. Franco believes in the theory that the best way to change traditional thinking is to make antiquated ideas obsolete through superior methodology. His innovative ideas have made a significant contribution to changing the thinking of many in the field about how people can best defend themselves against vicious and formidable adversaries.

Sammy Franco is perhaps best known as the founder and creator of Contemporary Fighting Arts (CFA), a state-of-the-art offensive-based combat system that is specifically designed for real-world self-defense. CFA is a sophisticated and practical system of self-defense, designed specifically to provide efficient and effective methods to avoid, defuse, confront, and neutralize both armed and unarmed attackers.

After studying and training in numerous martial art systems

and related disciplines and acquiring extensive firsthand experience from real "street" combat, Mr. Franco developed his first system, known as Analytical Street Fighting. This system, which was one of the first practical "street fighting" martial arts, employed an unrestrained reality-based training methodology known as Simulated Street Fighting. Analytical Street Fighting served as the foundation for the fundamental principles of Contemporary Fighting Arts and Mr. Franco's teaching methodology.

CFA also draws from the concepts and principles of numerous sciences and disciplines, including police and military science, criminal justice, criminology, sociology, human psychology, philosophy, histrionics, kinesics, proxemics, kinesiology, emergency medicine, crisis management, and human anatomy.

Sammy Franco has frequently been featured in martial art magazines, newspapers, and appeared on numerous radio and television programs. Mr. Franco has also authored numerous books, magazine articles and editorials, and has developed a popular library of instructional videos.

As a matter of fact, his book Street Lethal was one of the first books ever published on the subject of reality based self-defense. His other books include Killer Instinct, When Seconds Count, 1001 Street Fighting Secrets, First Strike, The Bigger They Are – The Harder They Fall, War Machine, War Craft, Ground War, Warrior Wisdom, Out of the Cage, Gun Safety Handbook, Heavy Bag Training, The Body Complete Body Opponent Bag, and Kubotan Power.

Sammy Franco's experience and credibility in the combat sciences is unequaled. One of his many accomplishments in this field includes the fact that he has earned the ranking of a Law Enforcement Master Instructor, and has designed, implemented, and taught officer survival training to the United States Border Patrol (USBP). He instructs members of the US Secret Service, Military Special Forces, Washington DC Police Department, Montgomery County, Maryland Deputy Sheriffs, and the US Library of Congress Police. Sammy Franco is also a member of the prestigious

International Law Enforcement Educators and Trainers Association (ILEETA) as well as the American Society of Law Enforcement Trainers (ASLET) and he is listed in the "Who's Who Director of Law Enforcement Instructors."

Sammy Franco is a nationally certified Law Enforcement Instructor in the following curricula: PR-24 Side-Handle Baton, Police Arrest and Control Procedures, Police Personal Weapons Tactics, Police Power Handcuffing Methods, Police Oleoresin Capsicum Aerosol Training (OCAT), Police Weapon Retention and Disarming Methods, Police Edged Weapon Countermeasures and "Use of Force" Assessment and Response Methods.

Mr. Franco is also a National Rifle Association (NRA) instructor who specializes in firearm safety, personal protection and advanced combat pistol shooting.

Mr. Franco holds a Bachelor of Arts degree in Criminal Justice from the University of Maryland. He is a regularly featured speaker at a number of professional conferences, and conducts dynamic and enlightening seminars on numerous aspects of self-defense and personal protection.

Mr. Franco has instructed thousands of students in his career, including instruction on street fighting, grappling and ground fighting, boxing and kick boxing, knife combat, multiple opponent survival skills, stick fighting, and firearms training. Having lived through street violence himself, Mr. Franco's goal is not its glorification, but to help people free themselves from violence and its costly price.

For more information about Mr. Franco and his unique Contemporary Fighting Arts system, you can visit his website at: www.sammyfranco.com

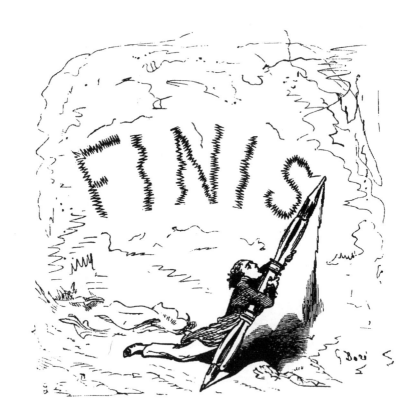

If you liked this book, you will also want to read these:

THE COMPLETE BODY OPPONENT BAG BOOK
by Sammy Franco

In this one-of-a-kind book, world-renowned martial arts expert, Sammy Franco teaches you the many hidden training features of the body opponent bag that will improve your fighting skills and accelerate your fitness and conditioning. Develop explosive speed and power, improve your endurance, and tone, and strengthen your entire body. With detailed photographs, step-by-step instructions, and dozens of unique workout routines, The Complete Body Opponent Bag Book is the authoritative resource for mastering this lifelike punching bag. 8.5 x 5.5, soft cover, photos, illustrations, 206 pages.

WAR MACHINE
How to Transform Yourself Into A Vicious & Deadly Street Fighter
by Sammy Franco

War Machine is a book that will change you for the rest of your life! When followed accordingly, War Machine will forge your mind, body and spirit into iron. Once armed with the mental and physical attributes of the War Machine, you will become a strong and confident warrior that can handle just about anything that life may throw your way. In essence, War Machine is a way of life. Powerful, intense, and hard. 11 x 8.5, soft cover, photos, illustrations, 210 pages.

OUT OF THE CAGE
A Complete Guide to Beating a Mixed Martial Artist on the Street
by Sammy Franco

Forget the UFC! The truth is, a street fight is the "ultimate no holds barred fight" often with deadly consequences, but you don't need to join a mixed martial arts school or become a cage fighter to defeat a mixed martial artist on the street. What you need are solid skills and combat proven techniques that can be applied under the stress of real world combat conditions. Out of the Cage takes you inside the mind of the MMA fighter and reveals all of his weaknesses, allowing you to quickly exploit them to your advantage. 10 x 7, soft cover, photos, illustrations, 194 pages.

CONTEMPORARY FIGHTING ARTS, LLC
"Real World Self Defense Since 1989"
www.sammyfranco.com
301-279-2244

Printed in Poland
by Amazon Fulfillment
Poland Sp. z o.o., Wrocław